Measuring Walking:
A Handbook of
Clinical Gait Analysis

Measuring Walking: A Handbook of Clinical Gait Analysis

Richard Baker

Professor of Clinical Gait Analysis,
University of Salford, Manchester, UK

Mac Keith Press
2013

© 2013 Mac Keith Press

Editor: Hilary M. Hart
Managing Director: Ann-Marie Halligan
Production Manager: Udoka Ohuonu
Project Manager: Ushadevi Medapati

The views and opinions expressed herein are those of the author and do not necessarily represent those of the publisher.

First published in this edition in 2013 by Mac Keith Press
2nd Floor, Rankin Building, 139-143 Bermondsey Street, London SE1 3UW
Reprinted 2018, 2020

British Library Cataloguing-in-Publication data
A catalogue record for this book is available from the British Library

ISBN: 978-1-908316-66-0

Typeset by Datamatics Global Services Limited

Printed by Ashford Colour Press Ltd, Gosport, Hampshire, UK

I dedicate this book to Oli, Abi and Melanie who have had to put up with so much because of their Dad's career. I'm so proud of all three of you.

Contents

All chapters have been written in consultation with Michael Schwartz

Contents

About the Author

Richard Baker is Professor of Clinical Gait Analysis at the University of Salford, Manchester, UK. He has spent nearly 20 years delivering or managing clinical gait analysis services. For nine years he was Manager of the Hugh Williamson Gait Analysis Service at the Royal Children's Hospital in Melbourne, Australia. During that time he served as Founding Director of the NHMRC Centre of Clinical Research Excellence in Gait Analysis and Gait Rehabilitation. He is currently developing a Joint European Master's Degree programme in Clinical Movement Analysis with colleagues in Belgium and the Netherlands. He writes a blog at www.wwrichard.net.

Acknowledgements

This book represents the result of over 25 years of working in the field alongside a whole range of wonderful people. Nine years of this were spent working at the Royal Children's Hospital and Murdoch Childrens Research Institute in Melbourne. This book embodies a culmination of that experience and documents how clinical gait analysis is conducted there (with a couple of minor variations). It was an output listed on the original grant application which led to the establishment of the Australian Medical Research Council's Centre of Clinical Research Excellence in Clinical Gait Analysis and Gait Rehabilitation.

Specific chapters have been written in consultation with some of my co-workers in Melbourne: Fiona Dobson, Adrienne Harvey, Jenny McGinley, Jill Rodda and Pam Thomason. Adam Shortland, ('Dr Muscles' as far as clinical gait analysis is concerned), has performed a similar role in relation to the chapters on electromyography. Alberto Leardini and Julie Stebbins have also provided comments on specific sections of Chapter 4. To maintain a consistent narrative voice, I have done the writing and they have done the commenting. The chapters are grounded in the experience I have gained from working with them before ever conceiving of this book and I want to acknowledge this as well as specific comments they have made on my drafts. Mike Schwartz willingly took on the role of consulting editor, which has required him to read and comment on each chapter as it was produced. There were relatively few areas where we differed which, given how much I respect his understanding of the field, gives me considerable confidence in the final product. The final editorial decisions were mine and I thus accept the responsibility for any shortcomings.

The book also reflects important but less direct influences on my thinking and career. David Condie was particularly influential in my first appointment at the Dundee Limb Fitting Centre and through him I claim a lineage to the classical biomechanics pioneered at Strathclyde University by Professor John Paul. At the Musgrave Park Hospital, I learnt alongside Aidan Cosgrove, Catherine Duffy, Sheila McNeill and Brona McDowell.

Professor Kerr Graham recruited me to Melbourne and his drive to deliver paediatric services of the very highest quality has been a continual inspiration to me. I take considerable pride in having been able to contribute towards those excellent services that he continues to provide to the children of Victoria. Having already acknowledged the Melbourne staff who contributed to specific chapters, I must also thank Adrienne Fosang, Tandy Hastings-Ison, Meg Morris, Marcus Pandy, Morgan Sangeux, Anthony Schache, Paulo Selber, Oren Tirosh and Rory Wolfe for numerous conversations and occasional arguments during which my knowledge and opinions have been forged. No less important have been a still growing list of students that I have supervised but who have also taught me.

I have grown up embedded in a family of clinical gait analysts on both sides of the Atlantic and in Australia. Working in this field is made special by the involvement it requires with a wide range of biomechanists, surgeons, physiotherapists, orthotists, prosthetists and others, all working at the edges of their own fields and at the interface with others. It would be wrong to mention individuals, but I do want to celebrate the diversity and strength of this community.

Finally, I thank my wife and family for putting up with me, my career and this book. My PhD records 'thanks to Liz who married me and my PhD and can now have me to herself'. If only life were that simple. I wonder what the next project will be?

Foreword

All science is either physics or stamp collecting.

If you can't explain your physics to a barmaid it is probably not very good physics.

Quoted in *Rutherford at Manchester* (1962) JB Birks

Richard Baker is the first Professor of Clinical Gait Analysis at the University of Salford, Manchester, UK His 'Measuring Walking: A Handbook of Clinical Gait Analysis' is a major contribution to the field from an inspirational teacher and will deservedly be popular. Richard's background is in Physics (BA, Cambridge, 1985) and Biomechanics (Dundee, PhD, 1994) followed by 25 years immersed in the practical aspects of Clinical Gait Analysis. He has set up gait laboratories, re-configured service delivery, developed new reporting tools and templates and constantly strived for improvements in every aspect of the complex chain that is clinical gait analysis.

Richard was appointed as Service Manager of the Mitre Gait Analysis Laboratory, Musgrave Park Hospital in 1994. In 2001, we were fortunate to recruit Richard as Technical Director and Director of Research, at the Hugh Williamson Gait Laboratory, Royal Children's Hospital, Melbourne. He filled this post with distinction until 2010, including four very productive years as Director of the NHMRC Centre of Clinical Research Excellence in Gait Analysis and Gait Rehabilitation.

Richard has made many major contributions to the field of clinical gait analysis through his research and teaching. He has a passion for clinical gait analysis and the ability to communicate effectively with biomedical engineers, kinesiologists, physiotherapists, physicians and surgeons. As expected from a physicist, he has a rigorous understanding of mechanics and measurement. However, he is also an excellent communicator and his writing is a model of clarity. Richard has taught many courses in clinical gait analysis, in many parts of the world and is a sought-after keynote speaker and guest lecturer.

Richard brings his clarity of thinking and expression to this important new text. He has the requisite scientific background tempered with 25 years of practical experience of setting up the clinical gait analysis service in Belfast and reconfiguring the service at the Royal Children's Hospital in Melbourne. Richard wrote all 15 chapters of this eminently practical textbook, ensuring consistency and avoiding repetition. However, he has included important contributions from colleagues including Adam Shortland (Electromyography), Adrienne Harvey and Jill Rodda (Clinical Video), Pam Thomason and Jill Rodda (Physical Examination) and the combined efforts of Jenny McGinley, Fiona Dobson and Pam Thomason in a crucial chapter on Interpretation and Reporting. New tools developed by Richard and his colleagues are described, including the Gait Profile Score, the Movement Analysis Profile and Gait Variable Scores. These are wonderful new tools for reporting gait studies, for change after intervention and in outcome studies.

Richard is acutely aware of the historical background to gait analysis, from Aristotle to Jurg Baumann and the crucial contributions from the North American pioneers, Jaquelin Perry, David Sutherland and Jim Gage. This does not stop him from challenging conventional wisdom, and only time will tell if his description of the phases of the gait cycle will replace the current convention.

He has strongly held views on the reliability of gait analysis and the need to separate this issue from the lack of agreement on treatment recommendations. Now that he works in a university setting rather than a clinical environment, he champions 'impairment based reporting' rather than the traditional Melbourne report which concludes with management options.

Who should buy this book and who should read it? I think it is a book, which should be front and centre, in every gait laboratory. It should be in the possession of all gait laboratory staff, from all professional backgrounds. It would be ideal preparatory reading before attending a course in clinical gait analysis and an excellent reference to retain thereafter. It will be very useful to the many clinical researchers, whose work brings them in contact with clinical gait analysis.

We the clinician/stamp collectors are grateful that Richard has made such a successful effort to communicate the essence of clinical gait analysis in this most practical and readable textbook. He has clearly passed Rutherford's test of being able to explain his physics to a barmaid.

Kerr Graham
The Hugh Williamson Gait Analysis Laboratory,
Royal Children's Hospital, Melbourne, Australia,
January 2013.

Reference

Birks JB. *Rutherford at Manchester*. New York: WA Benjamin Inc.,1962.

Preface

I passionately believe that if we can understand why patients walk the way they do then we will be able to help them walk better. Understanding how they walk will, in turn, be based on an understanding of why some of us without neuromusculoskeletal impairment walk the way we do. Whether we are considering people with or without impairments the understanding must be based on measurements. As Lord Kelvin, a product of Belfast, the city in which I first learnt to be a clinical gait analyst, put it:

> *I often say that when you can measure what you are speaking about, and express it in numbers, you know something about it; but when you cannot measure it, when you cannot express it in numbers, your knowledge is of a meagre and unsatisfactory kind; It may be the beginning of knowledge, but you have scarcely in your thoughts advanced to the state of science, whatever the matter may be.*
>
> (Thomson 1889)

Clinical gait analysis is, essentially, the process of making those measurements. The aim of this book is to describe that process. It is based on 20 years of experience of performing clinical gait analysis and of managing clinical gait analysis services. There is no doubt it will be of most interest and use to those involved in making measurements of walking in the context of clinical gait analysis. It should also be useful to clinicians who use the data. It will also contain much that will be useful to those measuring walking, running or other activities for other purposes.

Richard Baker
Manchester, UK
Februrary 2013

Reference

Thomson W. *Electrical units of measurement. Popular Lectures and Addresses, vol. 1.* London: MacMillan and Co, 1889.

Terminology

One of the issues of working in an interdisciplinary field is that terminology is adopted from a number of sources. There are therefore often multiple words for very similar, but not necessarily identical, concepts. People with a background in one discipline are sometimes unaware of the technical definitions of words arising within different disciplines and thus language is often used imprecisely. Concerns about the use of appropriate language further complicate the picture. It is, however, impossible to think, write or speak clearly about a patient without having a clear language to think, write and speak in. I have therefore tried to adopt a consistent terminology throughout this book. This chapter outlines the reasons for adopting some of these terms.

Simple English words have generally been preferred, but where specific technical terms are required these have been used. The common English word *walking* is preferred to the more technical term *gait* unless established practice is so strong that this would sound ridiculous as in *clinical gait analysis*. The person performing a gait analysis will be referred to as the *analyst* and the person being analysed simple as the *patient* or *person*. Although some people dislike the term 'patient', this avoids the use of the even more objectionable term *subject* or a variety of more generic terms that are often ambiguous. *Normal* and *abnormal* are not used to describe people but are used in relation to gait patterns and data relating to them. A normal gait pattern is that of people with no specific neuromusculoskeletal pathology. It is generally represented by average data and some representation of the variability around this. *Feature* is used for an aspect of an individual's gait data that differs from the normal data in some way. I tend to distinguish between gait *variables* that differ across the gait cycle and gait *parameters* that do not but acknowledge that this is personal usage.

Gait analysis *service* is preferred to gait analysis *laboratory* unless the reference is actually to the room in which the analysis is conducted. This serves as a reminder that clinical gait analysis is, first and foremost, a clinical service and not just a room full of complex measuring equipment. A *session* is an occasion on which a person visits a gait analysis service (an alternative word might be *appointment*). A single episode of data collection is a *trial*, which may be a *static* trial for patient *calibration* or a *walking* trial. A *condition* is the combination of factors that are similar for some number of trials such as the combination of orthoses and footwear, or whether sticks of crutches are being used. Some conditions require replacement of markers (e.g. in shoes or barefoot) in which case a separate calibration will be required, whereas others (e.g. walking with or without crutches) do not.

Anatomical planes are referred to as *sagittal*, *coronal* and *transverse* but are always related to a specific body segment. There is some ambiguity with these terms at the foot, but in this book *transverse* will still refer to the plane that separates top from bottom and *coronal* for the plane that separates front from back. Reference is also made to global planes – the *global sagittal* plane includes the vertical and the direction in which the person is asked to walk, the *global transverse* plane is the horizontal plane and the *global coronal* plane is perpendicular to both.

Movement of the hip and knee joints is described as *flexion*, *adduction* and *internal rotation*. Pelvic movements are described as *tilt* (sagittal plane, anterior is positive), *obliquity* (transverse plane, up is positive) and *rotation* (transverse plane, forward is positive). There is general consensus on the use of *dorsiflexion* to describe foot and ankle movement but not for other terms. In this book, *inversion* is rotation about the long axis of the foot and *adduction* is movement of that long axis out of the sagittal plane (*supination* is rarely used but refers to rotation about an axis oblique to the primary anatomical planes). All these terms should generally be read to include the opposite movements as negative values to avoid having to use clumsy expressions such as *flexion–extension* or *ab/adduction*. Precise definitions of relevant joint angles are given in Chapter 2. All these terms refer to movements of the joints; Latinised words (e.g. *varus*, *valgus*, *equinus* and *calcaneus*) are reserved for fixed deformities.

The terminology used to describe neurological signs is particularly complex with little consensus even among clinical neurologists. It is perhaps fortunate that our understanding of how different neurological features affect walking is still extremely superficial. A simple distinction will be adopted between *spasticity* representing neurological signs associated with movement (velocity dependent) and *tone* representing neurological signs present at rest.

Chapter 1

Introduction

Historical introduction

To understand contemporary clinical gait analysis it is useful to briefly review its history (Baker 2007). At least since the time of Aristotle (384–322BC) walking has fascinated scientists. Through the Renaissance and Enlightenment there became an increasing appreciation that human movement is regulated by the same underlying principles that govern the movement of inanimate objects, and the field of biomechanics began to emerge. Until the middle of the 19th century there was no way to record human movement, and most of the understanding of walking was essentially conjecture. The advent of photography, however, presented a means of making such measurements and allowed the first genuinely scientific attempts to understand walking. Pioneering work by Muybridge (1830–1904) and Marey (1830–1904) came to full fruition in the remarkable achievements of Braune (1831–1892) and Fischer (1861–1917) just before the turn of the 20th century.

The need to rehabilitate amputees returning from war stimulated both Amar (1879–1935) and Inman (1905–1980) to apply the new techniques to study walking in disabled populations and develop the first clinical research programmes to use movement analysis techniques. Reliance on laborious processes for both making measurements and processing data effectively prevented the application of the new techniques to the assessment of individual patients. The first such technique to become clinically practical was electromyography (EMG) and this was adopted by the early pioneers of clinical gait analysis, Perry (1918–2013), Sutherland (1923–2006) and Baumann (1926–2000). All three found it difficult to interpret the results without some understanding of how the patient was moving however. Perry developed semi-objective observational scales whilst Sutherland and Baumann developed movie-based techniques. Sutherland pushed further and started to develop techniques to abstract kinematic variables from cine film. Without automated data capture, however, these remained impractical in a clinical context.

The breakthrough came with the development of the video camera and of computers capable of processing the data that these produced. James Gage drove the team that pioneered the application of this new technology and opened the first modern clinical gait analysis service at the Newington Children's Hospital, Connecticut, USA in 1981. At around the same time several systems became commercially available and a number of hospitals in North America and Europe started developing similar services. It was not long before systems started incorporating force plate data and EMG recordings with the kinematic data extracted from the video signal.

Through the rest of the 20th century a broad consensus developed among this small group of clinical services on how to perform a clinical gait analysis. This tradition might appropriately be called *conventional* clinical gait analysis. Gage's commitment to promote clinical gait analysis and develop training and education packages was an important driver of this as was the rather inflexible VICON Clinical Manager software developed by a major commercial supplier of gait analysis systems. As the technology became more widely available in the early years of this century a large number of hospitals developed services using systems from a variety of suppliers with software that could be used more flexibly. A large number of sources for training and education have also been developed. The result is that whilst there is still a considerable degree of uniformity among the older, more established services, particularly in the US and UK, there is also considerable variability as to how clinical gait analysis is implemented amongst many of the newer services. Whilst there is much to be gained by experimenting with new approaches, constructive progress is most likely to be made by doing so within a thorough understanding of the conventional approach. The primary aim of this book is to provide an understanding at a level that gives clear guidance on how clinical gait analysis services can be delivered within this tradition.

What is clinical gait analysis?
Many of us involved in this field are so familiar with the use of complex measurement systems that we forget that for the vast majority of clinicians gait analysis is an observational process. This book, however, is essentially about instrumented gait analysis. Hereafter the term *instrumented* has been dropped simply because it is too cumbersome to be used repeatedly. There is a chapter on how to take a clinical video but the use of this is discussed primarily in relation to how this supplements data from more complex systems.

Many of the centres in which clinical gait analysis services were pioneered ran highly integrated services, typically in paediatric orthopaedics, in which the gait analysis was just one component. In these the boundary between performing a clinical gait analysis and treating the patient was often blurred or even non-existent. In other places the gait analysis is much more clearly delineated from clinical decision-making with one group of professionals performing the assessments and another making the decisions. Different models of service provision lead to different understandings of what clinical gait analysis actually is.

This book will assume that gait analysis is the process of determining what is causing patients to walk the way they do. This is based on instrumented measurement (which is an objective process) and a biomechanical interpretation of what these measurements mean (which still requires some subjectivity). Whilst this process can be used to inform clinical decision-making, it is possible to make a clear distinction from it. Gait analysis is sometimes referred to as diagnostic but there are very few conditions in which gait analysis actually contributes significantly to the diagnosis. It is perhaps preferable to consider it as an assessment process.

The distinction between assessment and decision-making is important because gait analysis has come in for significant criticism over the years. As typified by Wright (2003), this has two strands. The first is that there is unacceptable measurement variability. This was a justifiable criticism 10 years ago (Noonan et al. 2003) but more recent work suggests that with appropriate quality assurance procedures acceptable measurement error is achievable (McGinley et al. 2009). The second is that gait analysis results in 'widely divergent treatment recommendations'. This is not a valid criticism of the clinical gait analysis as defined in the paragraph above. Two surgeons looking at the same radiograph will choose to manage a fracture differently. Their choice will depend on their personal experience and expertise and what facilities are available to them. The fact that they make different decisions does not make us question whether they should have used that radiograph as part of the decision-making process. Indeed, there is an expectation that they should use whatever data is available and relevant to guide their clinical practice.

The distinction between assessment and decision-making is also important for ensuring excellence in service provision. Making reliable measurements in gait analysis and providing rigorous biomechanical interpretation is extremely difficult. Both these processes require high levels of knowledge and expertise. It will be a very rare person who can provide these and the similar levels of knowledge and expertise that are required for clinical decision-making and patient management. Acceptable levels of clinical performance of gait analysis will only come through maintaining a focus on the gait analysis process itself. This can be a considerable challenge in centres in which the patient assessment, clinical decision-making and patient management are integrated. In these situations it is probably even more important to maintain a conceptual distinction between the assessment and decision-making processes than in centres where the two roles are organisationally and/or physically separate.

The distinction is also important when deciding who should staff gait analysis facilities and how they should be trained. The historical blurring of the assessment process, clinical decision-making and patient management in the pioneering centres led to the assumption that gait analysis should be delivered by the existing clinical staff (generally physiotherapists) with some additional training. Measurement theory and biomechanics are, however, not generally taught rigorously in clinical training programmes (core skills in physics and mathematics may not even be demanded as an entry requirement to clinical professions) and there are very few options for being taught these in-depth later. The resulting lack of expertise has generally been filled by recruiting additional staff who do have these skills but generally have poor understanding of the clinical issues or the skills to manage a patient or conduct a clinical assessment. This results in the expense of employing two professional staff neither of whom is properly qualified to perform the required role. Standards of clinical gait analysis would almost certainly rise if a new profession of *clinical gait analyst* was developed with the appropriate education and training to be competent in all aspects of the clinical gait analysis process.

The level of detail of this book is intended to be sufficient to summarise all of the key areas with which the clinical gait analyst should be familiar. In places this summary may be difficult to follow unless the analyst has some existing understanding of the underlying concepts which draw from a large number of disciplines including (but not limited to) anatomy, physiology, biomechanics and measurement theory. In that case they may need to refer to other more basic text books from the individual disciplines. In other places the summary may not appear specific enough and they will have to think quite carefully about how general principles can be applied in specific situations. Both of these limitations reinforce how difficult it is to perform high-quality clinical gait analysis and what demands it makes of the clinical gait analyst. Whilst challenging this should be welcomed as it is this that guarantees continued employment for those highly educated and experienced professionals who constitute the gait analysis workforce!

There has always been a symbiotic relationship between clinical service delivery and clinical research in gait analysis. In an emerging field this was essential to develop new techniques for data capture and analysis. As the field matures and we begin to understand more and more how clinical gait analysis should be performed, however, it is necessary to start to differentiate these activities. This is important because high-quality service delivery and research activity require quite different attitudes. Modern clinical services operate within a framework of clinical governance. This requires staff with clinical training and experience to deliver practice in line with well-defined protocols based on the established evidence base. Research, on the other hand, flourishes in an environment of experimentation that pushes practice beyond that evidence base. The first responsibility of any modern clinical gait analysis service is to ensure the delivery of standardised evidence-based measurement services to patients. The aim of this book is to describe how to do this. Much of the detail, however, will also be of use to those interested in clinical research, particularly those who want to use established technologies in different research applications.

Gait analysis and cerebral palsy
The pioneering clinical gait analysis services that first made use of kinematic and kinetic measurements all worked with children with cerebral palsy. The early focus was

on assessing children for complex orthopaedic surgery and this has been extended to include other interventions such as selective dorsal rhizotomy, injections of botulinum toxin and prescription of orthoses. There has been a strong historical relationship between developments in clinical gait analysis and the care of the ambulant child with cerebral palsy.

Although patients with cerebral palsy are probably still the only group where there is reasonably widespread agreement in how and why clinical gait analysis should be conducted, a growing number of centres are starting to apply the techniques more widely. In a recent informal survey of European gait analysis services less than 50% of appointments were for children with cerebral palsy or similar conditions. Gait analysis for other conditions is a rapidly growing field, and there is no doubt that over coming years clinical gait analysis will come to be less automatically identified with cerebral palsy than it is at present.

The conventional approach to clinical gait analysis that this book aims to describe emerged within the pioneering centres that were focusing on children with cerebral palsy. Most of the key chapters are simply about good measurement practice and although methods were originally developed for use in one patient group they are generally applicable across all patient groups. The major exception to this is the chapter on physical examination which is focused on a paediatric neuromusculoskeletal assessment. Those working in different fields will need to modify this to reflect their own requirements. They should remain alert for other areas in which the requirements of their own particular practice might differ from the methods outlined within this book.

Different aspects of clinical gait analysis

Defining gait analysis as the process of determining what is wrong with a patient is rather too vague for practical purposes. In this book it will be assumed that the more specific aim of gait analysis is to define what impairments are most likely to be affecting the patients' walking pattern. This will be referred to as *impairment-focused gait analysis*. Following World Health Organization's recommendations impairments are defined as *a problem in body structures or functions such as significant deviation or loss* (WHO 2001). Hip flexor contracture, persistent femoral anteversion, gastrocnemius spasticity and gluteus medius weakness are all impairments. Defining gait analysis in this way distinguishes it clearly from clinical decision-making. While there appears to be a small step between suggesting that a child's walking is affected by a hip flexion contracture and recommending that they should have a hip flexor release there is a considerable gulf conceptually (and medico-legally). This book assumes that the outcome of a clinical gait analysis is a description of the impairments most likely to affect walking ability.

As we have seen this maps onto the surgical decision-making processes and is particularly suited to orthopaedic management with children with cerebral palsy. Neither the orthopaedic surgeon nor anyone else (at present) can do anything to repair the brain damage that is the fundamental cause of cerebral palsy, but they are able to operate on secondary impairments that have developed as a consequence of the underlying condition. Orthopaedic surgery is limited to rectifying these impairments and being given a list of what these are likely to be by a gait analyst is extremely useful.

This information may be less useful in different contexts, particularly perhaps in areas where gait analysis has considerable potential but is not yet routinely used. In gait rehabilitation, for example, where simply removing the impairments is not possible, it might be far more useful to understand how patients are achieving function despite the impairments that are affecting them. Rehabilitation can then focus on augmenting existing compensatory strategies (or even suggesting new ones). This approach could then be referred to as *function-focused gait analysis*.

At present function-focused gait analysis is much less well developed than impairment-focused gait analysis. The impairment-focused approach is based primarily on the recognition of patterns in the data. Function-focused gait analysis is much more challenging in that it generally requires a much deeper knowledge of the underlying biomechanics and an ability to relate these to the functional requirements of walking. There are few contemporary gait analysts capable of delivering such analyses. The basic techniques for making measurements are the same regardless of which of these two approaches are adopted but in considering how data are interpreted this book will focus on the impairments-focused approach.

A little separate from either impairment- or function-focused gait analysis is the role of gait analysis in monitoring progress and documenting outcomes. Whilst documentation of outcomes within formal clinical trials is clearly the remit of clinical research, a very important role of routine clinical gait analysis services has always been to provide data to allow clinicians to reflect on how individual patients are progressing and particularly how they have responded to earlier interventions. This is important in the ongoing management of the individual patient but may be even more important in developing further the clinician's appreciation of how to manage other patients in the future. Clearly the fundamental requirement of using any measurement technique for this purpose is confidence that differences between measurements made on different occasions are a consequence of real changes in the patient and not simply of inconsistencies in how the measurements are made.

Whatever the application, the fundamental requirement of clinical gait analysis is for high-quality data that accurately and precisely record how the patient is walking. The fundamental purpose of this book is to describe how to provide such data. Even in a book of this length on what appears to be an extremely specific topic, however, it is only possible to do this at a rather general level. Individual analysts in individual clinical services will still need to adapt the general principles outlined to the specific requirements of their own professional practice.

References

Baker R The history of gait analysis before the advent of modern computers. *Gait Posture*, 2007, 26:331–342. DOI: 10.1016/j.gaitpost.2006.10.014

McGinley JL, Baker R, Wolfe R, Morris ME. The reliability of three-dimensional kinematic gait measurements: a systematic review. *Gait Posture*, 2009, 29:360–369. DOI: 10.1016/j.gaitpost.2008.09.003

Noonan K, Halliday S, Browne R, O'Brien S, Kayes K. Inter-observer variability of gait analysis in patients with cerebral palsy. *J Pediatr Orthop*, 2003, 23:279–287.

World Health Organization *International Classification of Functioning, Disability and Health*. World Health Organization, 2001.

Wright J. Pro: Interobserver variability of gait analysis. *J Pediatr Orthop*, 2003, 23:288–289.

Chapter 2

Basic measurements

The power of gait analysis rests in the concept of the *gait cycle*. Walking is achieved by moving the body in a particular manner to make a stride with more or less similar movements and then repeating this on an ongoing basis. The series of movements that is repeated is referred to as a gait cycle. Each gait cycle can be taken as representative of how a person walks, and comparison of a number of cycles can be taken as an indication of how variable that pattern is. Gait analysis is based on an assumption that this cyclic motion is an important indicator of locomotor function. Attempts to extend gait analysis to other types of movements, such as upper extremity movement, are far less powerful because the functional requirement is often not achieved by cyclic activity and 'inventing' cyclic activities simply to allow measurements to be made is far less clinically relevant.

Spatial parameters[1]

At its most fundamental, the gait cycle is a pattern of movement in which the feet are moved forwards alternately while the rest of the body moves forwards over these. A *step* is the movement of one foot in front of the other. A *stride* is made up of a step for one foot followed by another step for the other (Figure 2.1). By almost universal convention, the gait cycle is taken to start at the instant that one foot makes contact with the floor, *foot contact*, and continuing until the next occasion when the same foot makes contact with the floor again. (In healthy walking, it is the heel that contacts the ground first and this instant is often referred to as heel-strike. If we want a terminology that can be used for all

---

[1] In this book, gait *parameters* will be used to refer to quantities defined for a whole gait cycle or part of it. Gait *variables* will refer to quantities that vary continuously through the gait cycle.

patients, including those who do not make first contact with the heel, *foot contact* is the preferred term.)

Step length is the distance that one part of the foot travels in front of the same part of the other foot during each step. *Stride length* is the distance that one part of a foot travels between the same instant in two consecutive gait cycles. It does not actually matter which instant is chosen, but it is very common to use foot contact. Given that during a stride the left foot moves in front of the right by right step length and the right then moves in front of the left by left step length, then it can be seen that stride length must be the sum of left and right step lengths. On average, the stride length for one side must be the same as that for the other (otherwise the person will not be walking in a straight line) regardless of how asymmetric other aspects of the gait pattern may be. In asymmetric gait patterns, however, the step lengths for the two sides may be different (Figure 2.2).

Step width is a measure of the mediolateral separation of the feet. Specific definitions of the term vary quite considerably in the literature. What is certain is that step width is really a function of the stride (it is the same for left and right steps) and that *stride width* should be the preferred term. It can be seen from Figure 2.3 that step width will depend on the point on the foot used as the basis of measurement. The distance between the heels is a commonly used measure that can easily be measured from video or foot prints. In a three-dimensional gait analysis, the distance between the ankle joint centres is probably the most useful definition.

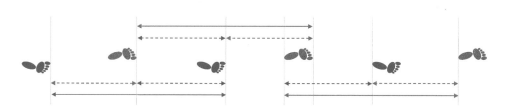

Figure 2.1 Step (---) and stride (—) lengths for symmetrical walking.

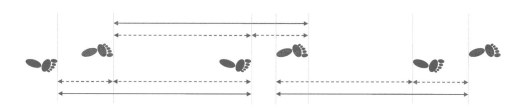

Figure 2.2 Step (---) and stride (—) lengths for asymmetrical walking.

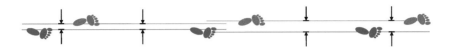

Figure 2.3 Stride width. Note that 'step widths' for left and right sides are identical regardless of any asymmetry in the gait pattern but that the size of step width depends on whether the heel (left) or middle of fore-foot (right) is chosen as the basis for measurement.

Temporal parameters

Stride time is the duration of one gait cycle. As with stride length, it does not really matter which point of the gait cycle it is calculated from, but by convention it is taken as the time between successive foot strikes on the same side. It is far more common, however, to refer to the duration of the gait cycle indirectly through specifying the *cadence*. This is the number of cycles taken in a specified time. There is some variability in the literature as to how to describe the number of cycles (steps or strides) and the time interval (seconds or minutes). The most common practice is probably to use steps per minute. This will, of course, be twice the number of strides per minute, and this difference is generally sufficiently large that there is little ambiguity in which convention is being used (though care may be needed for particularly slow walkers). *Step time* is sometimes defined analogously to stride time particularly when measures of gait symmetry are useful. Occasionally left or right side *cadence* is defined as the reciprocal of left or right step time; this is extremely misleading (cadence is only meaningful if defined for a stride) and is a practice best avoided.

Walking speed, the distance travelled in a given time, is related to both cadence and stride length:

$$\text{Walking speed} = \frac{\text{cadence} \times \text{stride length}}{120}$$

where walking speed is in metres/second, cadence is in steps per minute and stride length is in metres. If measurements are in different units then the number 120 needs to be changed accordingly. It can be argued that there is little point, given this mathematical relationship, for quoting all three measurements, but it can be clinically useful to think of walking speed as being determined by the other two parameters. Therefore, one patient might be described as walking slowly as a consequence of reduced step length but normal cadence whereas another might be described as walking at normal speed by increasing cadence to compensate for a short step length.

Phases of gait

In order to describe the processes that occur during walking, it is useful to divide the gait cycle into a number of phases. The simplest such division is to divide the cycle for a given limb into the stance phase, when the foot is in contact with the floor, and the swing phase, when it is not. In healthy walking at comfortable speed, this happens about 60% into the gait cycle (some studies suggest that 62% is a closer estimate). The point at which stance ends is *foot off* (often referred to as toe-off).

To develop this scheme by further subdividing the gait cycle, it is possible to depict what is happening to the other leg at the same time (see Figure 2.5). If the walking pattern is symmetrical, then the *opposite foot contact* will occur half-way through the gait cycle. *Opposite foot off* (from the preceding gait cycle) precedes this by the duration of the opposite swing phase (approximately 40% of the cycle in normal walking). This subdivides stance into *first double support* (from foot contact to opposite foot off), *single support* (from opposite foot off to opposite foot contact) and *second double support* (from opposite foot contact to foot off) (see Figure 2.5).

Single support and swing are both long phases, and further subdivision is useful. Such subdivision is essentially arbitrary. The most widely accepted scheme for subdivision is that proposed by Perry (1992), but there are several problems with this (described in the Appendix 1) and a simple division of both single support and swing into three subphases of equal duration and referred to as *early*, *middle* and *late* will be used in this book (see Figure 2.6).

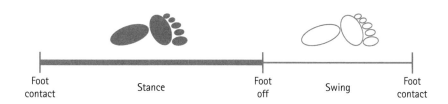

Figure 2.4 A single stride divided into stance and swing phases.

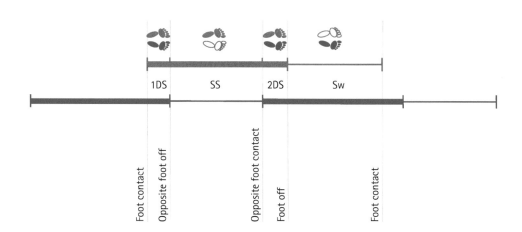

Figure 2.5 Subdivision of a gait cycle into periods of double and single support on the basis of events occurring on the opposite limb.

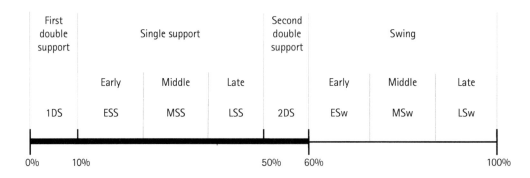

Figure 2.6 The phases of the gait cycle based on equal subdivision of single support and swing into three phases.

Gait graphs

Gait variables, quantities that vary throughout the gait cycle, are plotted on gait graphs. The gait graph (see Figure 2.7) has time, in percentage of the gait cycle, plotted along the horizontal axis and the gait variable plotted on the vertical axis. By convention, reference data are expressed as one standard deviation ranges. It is important to remember that 35% of reference data fall outside this range, and it is useful to plot the two standard deviation range in a different shade of grey (only 2% of data fall outside this). Gait variables are plotted in different colours, and throughout this book data from the left side will be plotted in red and from the right in blue.[2] Foot off for both sides are plotted as vertical lines across the full height of the graph in the appropriate colours. Opposite foot off and opposite foot contacts are plotted as tick marks across the top of the graph (sometimes across the bottom).

With such colour coding, it is quite possible to over-plot data from several trials. This is probably the most useful procedure for the experienced gait analyst as it allows a comparison of the pattern and the consistency of the traces at the same time. Although over-plotting too many traces can make it difficult to distinguish the characteristics of individual traces, somewhere between four and seven traces are probably most useful. The practice of selecting a 'representative trial' was largely a requirement imposed by less flexible graphing software in the past. It may be misleading, particularly as a trial that is representative for one variable may not be representative for others. It is inappropriate if such data are to be used in formal statistical analyses and should generally be avoided.

_____

[2] This convention reflects western European politics in which left-wing parties tend to adopt the colour red and right-wing parties adopt the colour blue. The other obvious convention to follow is a nautical convention with left (port) in red and right (starboard) in green. Unfortunately this can be problematic for people with red–green colour blindness.

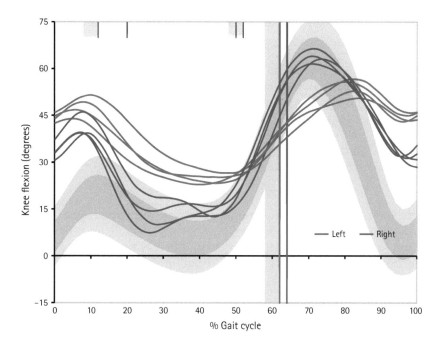

Figure 2.7 Standard gait graph for knee flexion with reference data for one standard deviation (darker grey) and two standard deviations (lighter grey). Note that there are subtle features during mid-stance on the right (blue) side that might have been considered clinically important if any one trace had been chosen as 'representative' but, which over-plotting of several traces makes clear, are not a characteristic of the patient.

It is much easier to interpret data if graphs are always laid out in the same format. Two particular issues that should be standardised are the aspect ratio (ratio of height to width) and scaling of graphs. If either of these is changed, then the data can appear very different. The aspect ratio is the ratio of the height of the graph to its width. All graphs in this book will be plotted with an aspect ratio of 0.75 (3 units high to 4 units across). Different types of gait variables have different dimensions (measured in different units), and it is not sensible to standardise scaling for such different measures. It may be useful to standardise variables with similar dimensions, but because variables may vary in the range they span during walking this is not always possible. Most of the kinematic variables can be scaled from −30° to +30°. The exceptions are pelvic tilt (0° to 60°), hip flexion (−20° to 70°) and knee flexion (−15° to 75°). Note that using the overall range for pelvic tilt (60°) matches the other graphs and hip and knee flexion are plotted across the same overall range (90°).

It is important to remember that variables from each side are plotted with respect to gait cycles defined for the corresponding sides. The points plotted for the left and right side at the same instant in the gait cycle do not correspond to the same instant in real time.

The temporal relationship between data for left and right sides is illustrated in Figure 2.8. Traces for left and right knee angles over several gait cycles are plotted against the same timescale. Peak knee flexion occurs during swing for one side which corresponds to stance for the other. This has been marked by a dot on the traces. When the data from both sides are combined into one graph (bottom of Figure 2.8), the two dots appear at quite different time-points. The points are separated by approximately half a gait cycle. (They are actually separated by the time to opposite foot contact but this is generally close to half a gait cycle except in particularly asymmetric gait patterns.) In order to see what is happening on one leg at a particular point in the gait cycle for the other leg, it is necessary to look either approximately half a gait cycle forwards or backwards on the same graph.

Data interpretation is also much simpler if the graphs are always arranged in the same arrays (see Figure 2.9). It is almost universal for the rows in graph arrays to run from proximal (top) to distal (bottom). Most services plot transverse plane data in the right-hand column, but there is some inconsistency regarding sagittal and coronal plane measurements. In this book, sagittal plane data will always be plotted in the left-hand column. Some graphs are less clinically relevant and may be omitted (but it should also be noted that some graphs that have little clinical relevance may serve as indicators of data quality). Which these are may depend on the patient group.

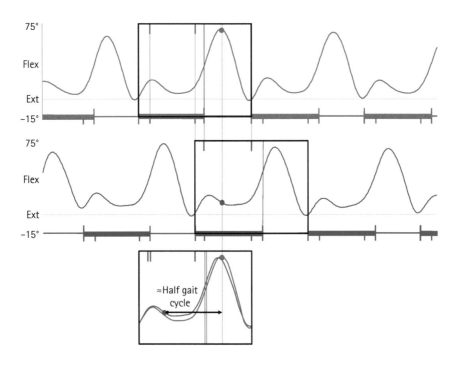

Figure 2.8 Temporal relationship between data for left and right sides.

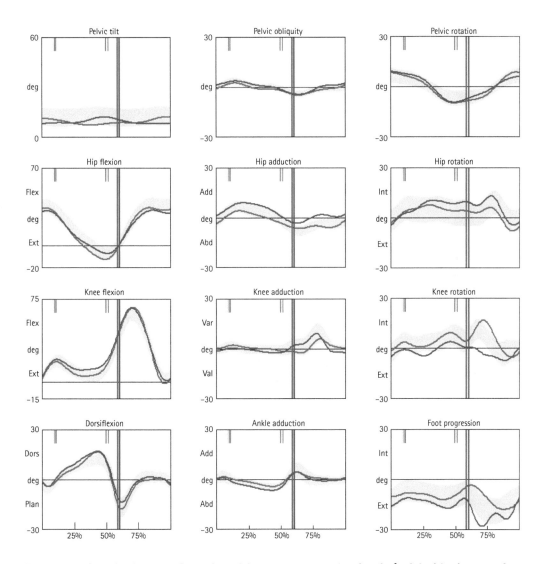

Figure 2.9 Standard array of graphs, with rows representing levels (pelvis, hip, knee and ankle) and columns representing planes (sagittal, coronal and transverse).

Kinematics

Kinematics describe the way the body moves. The human anatomy is extremely complex, and a comprehensive description of how all the body parts move is not possible; so we simplify things by considering a *model* of the body. This has multiple segments that can be described by referring either to the segment's major bone (e.g. pelvis, femur and tibia) or to some other name (e.g. foot, trunk and head). Each of these segments is assumed to be a rigid body (the segment itself does not change shape during walking). At any instant of time, the body will be in a specific configuration which is called a *pose*. In a *six degree of freedom* (6DoF) model, each of the segments is free both to translate and to rotate independently of the other segments. The pose of such a model then has to be described by the position and orientation of each of the segments. In an *articulated* model, the segments are assumed to be linked by joints, and these constrain the movement. The pose of such a model is then completely specified by the orientation of the segments. In practice, current measurement systems are not precise or accurate enough to measure segment translations well; so most clinical gait analysis is based on the interpretation of the joint angles only (regardless of whether a 6DoF or articulated model is used).

To understand exactly what the joint angles represent, it is necessary to consider each segment as having a *coordinate system* embedded within it, which allows its orientation to be described. In two dimensions, this can be depicted by two mutually perpendicular arrows or axes that are conventionally labelled *x* and *y* in approximately forward and upward directions, respectively (Wu and Cavanagh 1995; Wu et al. 2002). These are only approximate as the precise definitions depend on the model used and the orientation of the segment at the time the measurement is made. The model specifies how one of the axes, the *primary axis*, is defined from the anatomy of the segment and the other axis is, by definition, perpendicular to this. Therefore, for the most common sagittal plane model, the primary axis for the pelvis runs from the posterior superior iliac spine (PSIS) to the anterior superior iliac spine (ASIS, see Figure 2.10). For most people in standing or walking, this points forwards and downwards a little. The proximal axis is the arrow perpendicular to this. For the femur and tibia segments, the proximal axis is the primary axis running from the distal joint centre to the proximal joint centre and the anterior axis is the mutual perpendicular. For the foot, the anterior axis, running parallel to the plantar surface, is the primary axis and the proximal axis is perpendicular.

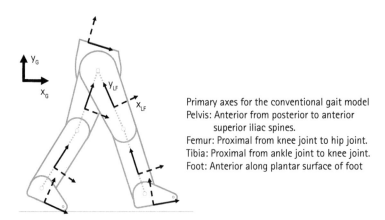

Primary axes for the conventional gait model
Pelvis: Anterior from posterior to anterior
  superior iliac spines.
Femur: Proximal from knee joint to hip joint.
Tibia: Proximal from ankle joint to knee joint.
Foot: Anterior along plantar surface of foot

Figure 2.10 Articulated seven-segment model to describe movement in the sagittal plane. Solid lines represent primary axes and dashed lines represent the perpendicular direction used to define the coordinate system. The *x* and *y* axes of the global (G) and left femur (LF) coordinate systems are labelled.

Segment kinematics describe the orientation of the segment with respect to some global coordinate system. This is almost always defined by a vertical axis (upwards) and a horizontal axis pointing in the direction of walking. The segment angle is then the angle between the same axes (x or y) of the segment and global coordinate systems. Joint kinematics describe the orientation of one segment with respect to an adjacent segment. For any joint, this is the angle between the same axes (x or y) for the two adjacent segments. The knee angle is the angle between either the x or y axes of the tibia and femur segments.

This approach needs a little modification for three-dimensional kinematics. The coordinate system is then comprised of three mutually perpendicular axes. The x and y axes are still broadly directed forwards and upwards and the z-axis to the side. It is still useful to consider one axis as primary. To define the secondary axis, we assume it is perpendicular to this but have to specify the plane in which it lies. By definition, the third axis is perpendicular to the first two axes and does not need to be defined explicitly. Exactly how the segment axes are defined will vary from one biomechanical model to another, and this is more fully described in Chapters 3 and 4. Once these axes have been defined, it is useful to consider them as describing anatomical planes for the segment. The plane containing the segment forward and upward axes is the segment sagittal plane, that containing the segment upward and lateral axes is the segment coronal plane and that defining the segment forward and lateral axes is the segment transverse plane (see Figure 2.11). In general, the anatomical planes for different segments do not align. To understand the nuances of gait analysis data, the analyst has to think in terms of these different segment anatomical planes.

To describe the relative orientation of two coordinate systems in three dimensions, three numbers are required and these are referred to as joint angles. For many purposes within clinical gait analysis it is sufficient simply to consider these as sagittal (generally flexion and extension), coronal (generally abduction and adduction) and transverse plane (internal and external rotation) joint angles. For understanding more subtle features in the data, however, it is important to know exactly how they are defined. Perhaps the clearest way to describe this is to use the globographic method (Strasser 1917; Dempster 1956; Pearl et al. 1992; Doorenbosch et al. 2003; Baker 2011). Using this system, the first two angles (generally flexion and abduction) describe the angles between the principle axis of the distal segment and that of the equivalent axis of the proximal segment described in terms of an imaginary globe superimposed in the proximal segment. These are analogous to the use of longitude and latitude. The third angle (internal rotation) represents rotation around the principle axis.[3]

Therefore, for the hip (Figure 2.12), flexion and abduction describe the alignment of the long axis of the femur with respect to the coronal and sagittal planes of the femur

---

[3] This is actually analogous to surface bearing (degrees from north) in navigation but the analogy is much less explicit than that of the first two angles to longitude and latitude and may therefore be less useful.

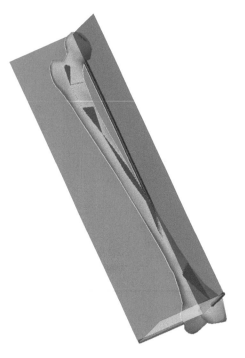

Figure 2.11 Definition of coordinate system for the femur for the conventional gait model. The primary (long) axis runs from the knee joint centre to the hip joint centre. The femur coronal plane (red) is the plane containing this primary axis and the line from this to the lateral epicondyle. The secondary axis (lateral) is in this plane and perpendicular to the long axis. The third axis (anterior) is perpendicular to the other two axes. The femur sagittal plane (blue) is that containing the anterior and long axes and the femur transverse plane (green) is that containing the anterior and lateral axes.

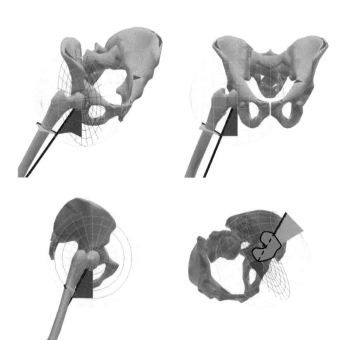

Figure 2.12 Joint angles for the hip joint (top left, three-dimensional view; top right, in coronal plane of femur; bottom left, in sagittal plane of femur; bottom right, looking along primary axis of femur). The thick black line is the primary (long) axis of the femur and the thinner line indicates internal and external rotation. The red angle indicates abduction (away from the equator). The blue angle represents extension (around the equator). The green angle represents external rotation about the primary axis.

respectively described in terms of a globe fixed in the femur. It has its centre at the hip joint and the equatorial plane lies parallel to the pelvis sagittal plane. Abduction is the angle between the primary axis of the femur and the sagittal plane. Flexion is the angle between the primary axis of the femur and coronal plane when projected onto the sagittal plane of the pelvis. Internal rotation is about the primary axis of the femur. Angles for the knee joint are described analogously, with the globe having its centre at the knee joint and its equatorial plane parallel to the femur sagittal plane.

Ankle angles are described analogously except that the primary axis of the foot is the anterior axis so dorsiflexion and abduction describe the position of the anterior axis of the foot with respect to the anterior axis of the tibia (Figure 2.13a). The primary axis of the pelvis (for lower body gait analysis) is the mediolateral axis (from one hip joint to the other, Figure 2.13b). For this reason, the orientation of the pelvis with respect to the global coordinate system is described in terms of a globe, with its equator lying in the horizontal plane (Baker 2001, 2011).

Kinetics

The ground reaction
Kinetics describe the forces and moments acting on and within the human body. It is these that cause the body to move in the way it does following the same laws of physics that govern the movement of other mechanical systems. Forces act to accelerate a body and do so independent of where the force is applied. A force is fully specified if we know its size (or magnitude) and the direction in which it is acting. This is most easily

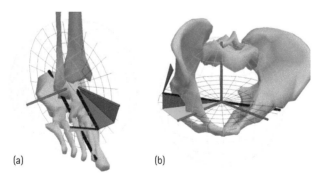

(a)   (b)

Figure 2.13 Ankle and pelvic angles. The primary axis of the foot passes through the ankle parallel to the long axis of the foot. Plantarflexion is illustrated in blue (round the equator), abduction in red (away from the equator) and inversion in green (around the primary axis). Pelvic angles are with respect to the global coordinate system (in red). Pelvic rotation (of primary axis around equator) is depicted in green, obliquity (away from equator) in red and anterior tilt (around primary axis) in blue.

visualised as an arrow, with its length representing the magnitude of the force. The most important force in gait analysis is the ground reaction,[4] which is the force exerted by the ground on the foot (see Figure 2.14). It is called a *reaction* because it is the equal and opposite force to that which the combination of gravity and muscle activity within the body exerts upon the ground. Although many gait analysis services do not even plot out the ground reaction, it is impossible to understand joint moments properly without a knowledge of how it is acting.

Whilst the ground reaction is most easily visualised as an arrow, it can only be plotted on gait graphs if we describe it in terms of individual components (Figure 2.14). In two dimensions, these are anterior and vertical, and these directions are always defined in the global coordinate system. In three dimensions, an additional mediolateral component is required. The vertical component is always positive (ground can only push the foot up – it cannot pull it down!), but the other two components may be positive or negative. The ground reaction supports the body against gravity and also accelerates the body's centre of mass. Resisting gravity takes much more force than accelerating the body during walking and running, so the vertical component of the ground reaction is always much larger than the other components.

Joint moments
Moments are similar to forces except they act to produce rotational accelerations (forces produce linear accelerations). Moments arise when a force is exerted at some distance from a joint. The further from the joint, the greater the moment generated for a given force. The total moment exerted by a force is the product of the magnitude of the force and the perpendicular distance of the force from the joint centre (Figure 2.14). The joint moments reported in clinical gait analysis are the total moment exerted by all the internal structures acting across any joint. If the joint is within its range of motion, then this moment is almost entirely attributable to the muscles acting across the joint.

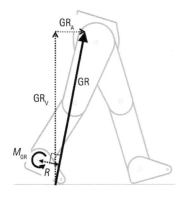

Figure 2.14 **The ground reaction at opposite foot contact. The reaction is most easily visualised as an arrow (solid, GR) but to be graphed it has to be described in terms of its anterior (GR$_A$) and vertical (GR$_V$) components (dotted). The moment the ground reaction exerts at the ankle (M_{GR}) is the product of the magnitude of the ground reaction and the perpendicular distance (R) from the ground reaction to the ankle joint centre.**

---

[4] Note that a *reaction* is a force, so there is no need to refer to ground reaction *force*.

Towards the end of the range of motion, stretching of ligaments and some resistance from bone geometry may also contribute to this moment.

This internal moment can be calculated from the measured ground reaction and the kinematics using a process called inverse dynamics, which takes account of the action of gravity and any acceleration on the body segments. This requires the acceleration and relative positions of the body segments to be determined from kinematic measurements and some estimates of the mass and moments of inertia of the body segments. These are generally based on the weight of the person and the lengths of the different segments as determined from the kinematics. Both the mass and moment of inertia of the foot and tibia are relatively small, and the internal ankle and knee moments are quite similar to the ground reaction moment at the respective joints. The effects of acceleration of the foot, tibia and femur on the hip moment, however, cannot be ignored. During normal walking, these are remarkably similar but opposite in magnitude to the effects of gravity on the body segments; so the internal hip moment is still quite similar to the ground reaction moment at the hip. This cannot be assumed for pathological gait, and full inverse dynamic calculations are always required if joint moments are going to be used for clinical gait analysis.

The way the body moves depends on the combined effect of all the moments acting at all the joints (Zajac and Gordon 1989). It is not possible to determine how an individual joint will move on the basis of the internal moment calculated for that joint alone. Therefore, just because there is an internal extensor moment at the knee it does not follow that the knee will necessarily extend. How the knee moves will depend on the moments at all the other joints as well. Indeed if this was not the case, then eccentric muscle activity would never occur. The only information that the internal joint moments gives is the net effect of the muscles acting across that joint (and of the ligaments or bones if the joint is at the end of its range of motion). If there is antagonistic activity in muscle groups, then the internal moment is the difference between the muscles acting in one sense (the extensors for example) and those acting in the other sense (the flexors). The joint moments indicate which are the dominant muscle groups acting at any given joint. They do not give any indication as to which individual muscles are acting within that group.

It is reasonably easy to develop an understanding of joint moments in two dimensions but, as with joint angles, more complex factors emerge in three dimensions. As with kinematics, these factors will have little effect on most clinical gait analysis but if subtle features in the data are of interest then a fuller understanding is required. A particular issue is that there are a number of conventions that can be used for plotting kinetic data, and different choices of these will lead to differences to the data (Schache and Baker 2007; Schache et al. 2007). These differences are generally quite small, and if the data are interpreted through comparison to reference data plotted using exactly the same conventions, then it is unlikely that these differences will affect any inferences made. On the other hand, if data plotted using different conventions are compared, then differences in the data may be large enough to mislead the gait analyst.

There is some confusion with the term *external moments*. Sometimes this is used to refer to the direct effect of the ground reaction at a joint (no use of inverse dynamics), and there is some sense in this terminology. In other times, it is used to refer to a full inverse dynamic calculation but represented in terms of the 'external moment' applied to the joint. An internal flexor moment is described as an external extensor moment. This is really quite misleading as the gravitational and inertial effects are not external. For these reasons, all moments in this book will be reported as *internal moments*.

Another issue relates to the coordinate system in which the moment is calculated. Most gait analysis softwares assume that an orthogonal coordinate system is most appropriate and allow the user to select between the global system or that of the proximal or distal segment (Figure 2.15). Given that all that the joint moments represent is the activity

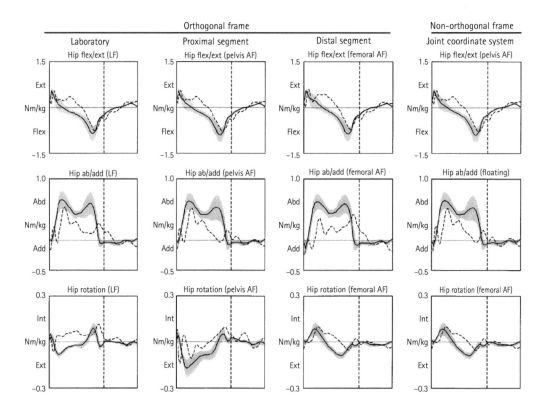

Figure 2.15 Ankle moments plotted with reference to different coordinate systems for a child with cerebral palsy and for a range of healthy adults (Figure from Schache and Baker 2007 with permission). Note marked differences particularly for rotational and inversion/eversion moments and also the reduced variability among healthy adults for the non-orthogonal frame.

of different muscle groups, it makes little sense to use the global coordinate system, but there is no particularly convincing argument for preferring one segment over the other. In this book, an arbitrary decision has been taken to represent all moments in an orthogonal coordinate system in the distal segment. Using an orthogonal axis system, however, means that the joint moments are incompatible with the joint angles. For example, an internal adductor moment will not generally be occurring about the same axis as the axis about which joint adduction angle is measured. It makes far more sense to describe joint moments about the same axes as the rotations are described (Schache and Baker 2007), and it is hoped that this will become the accepted convention in future. Schache and Baker also noted that this reduces the interindividual variability within the healthy population for some joint moments.

Joint powers
If the body is considered as consisting of a number of segments with a number of separate actuators (motors) acting at each joint instead of muscles, then the power that each actuator would have to supply is given by multiplying the joint angular velocity by the joint moment. This quantity is called the *joint power* and is often plotted out on gait graphs. The quantity is physically well defined, and patients often show joint powers that are different to normative data. These often correlate with the general aspects of the patient's condition, for example a patient with weak plantarflexors will often exhibit reduced ankle power. A detailed understanding of what the power data mean though is often quite difficult. Many of the most important muscles act over two or more joints, and the assumption of independent actuators acting at different joints is not a good model of how the body works. For example, in second double support energy is being generated at the hip but absorbed at the knee. If the rectus femoris is active, then it is quite possible that this represents a passive transfer of energy that gives the *appearance* of power generation at the hip and absorption at the knee (see Figure 2.16).

Normalisation
Clinical gait analysis is used for patients with a variety of body dimensions and mass. Normalisation is the processing of data in such a way as to try and reduce the effect of that variability on the underlying gait data. A heavy adult will be expected to exert a higher ground reaction than a young child. If we report data in units of total force (Newtons), it will be difficult to compare the data. If we divide the readings by body mass, however, then the resulting measurements (Newtons/kilogram) may be more comparable. Normalisation of data is very common in gait analysis.

Where the relationship between a measured variable and the size or mass of the individual is known, the normalisation schemes may be obvious. We know that force is almost always proportional to mass in mechanics; so dividing force measurements by body mass is sensible. With more complex variables, self-selected walking speed for example, it is not at all obvious how data should be normalised. *Non-dimensionalisation* can be used here to suggest appropriate methods. Most measurements have dimensions (units), and dividing these by a quantity with the same dimensions results in a quantity that is non-dimensional. Non-dimensional measurements are often less subject to

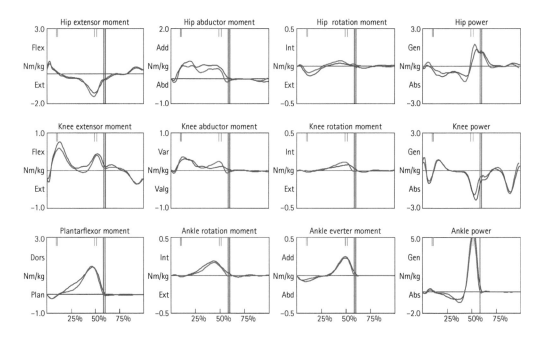

Figure 2.16 Joint moment and power data. Normal ranges (one standard deviation) and data from a single healthy person. Note that the ankle rotation moment and the hip, knee and ankle evertor moments are considerably smaller in magnitude than the other moments, and many clinical services choose not to plot these components.

variability with size. Stride length (with dimensions of length) divided by height (which also has dimensions of length) is likely to be less variable from person to person than the raw measure of stride length (in metres). Of course, some care is needed in deciding what to divide by; dividing stride length by waist circumference is likely to result in some very strange results despite it also being a length measurement. What can be said, however, is that data that have dimensions have probably not been normalised properly. It is very common to divide joint moments (Nm) by weight (N). The resulting quantity still has the units of metres, however, which should serve as a warning that moments depend on length as well as on weight and should be normalised by a length measurement as well as a weight measurement. Quite why this is not a standard practice in clinical gait analysis is unclear.

Alexander and Jayes (1983) took this approach further and proposed a dynamic similarity hypothesis which was summarised by Hof (1996) as a basis for normalisation of gait data and is becoming more and more widely accepted (see Table 2.1). This allows all common measurements to be scaled according to body mass (m_o), leg length (l_o) and the acceleration due to gravity (g) to make them non-dimensional in a manner consistent with the laws of dynamics. Whilst this is a

Table 2.1 Non-dimensional normalisation of gait analysis data

Quantity	Symbol	Dimension	Dimensionless number
Mass	M	M	$\hat{m} = \dfrac{m}{m_0}$
Length, distance	l, x	L	$\hat{l} = \dfrac{l}{l_0}$
Time	T	T	$\hat{t} = \dfrac{t}{\sqrt{l_0/g}}$
Speed, velocity	V	L T^{-1}	$\hat{v} = \dfrac{v}{gl_0}$
Force	F	M L T^{-2}	$\hat{F} = \dfrac{F}{m_0 g}$
Moment	M	M L^2 T^{-2}	$\hat{M} = \dfrac{M}{m_0 gl_0}$
Oxygen rate (per time)	R	M L^2 T^{-3}	$\hat{r} = \dfrac{r}{m_0 g\sqrt{gl_0}}$
Oxygen cost (per distance)	C	MLT^{-2}	$\hat{c} = \dfrac{c}{m_0 g}$

Angle is already a dimensionless quantity. m_0 is the body mass and l_0 is the leg length (Hof suggests greater trochanter to floor) and g is 9.81ms^{-2}. Note that for oxygen rate and cost, the oxygen volume needs to be converted to Joules (20.1J is equivalent to 1ml O$_2$) (Hof 1996).

sensible theoretical approach, it requires experimental validation; if the normalisation has been successful then the normalised variable should be independent of leg length or body mass. This has been established for walking speed (Vaughan et al. 2003) and oxygen cost and consumption (Schwartz et al. 2006) but has not been rigorously tested for other variables.

Normalisation may not always be appropriate. Take the example of a person with osteoarthritis of the knee which is exacerbated by the load exerted through the knee. If the person loses weight, then both the force and moment acting across the knee will be reduced (probably in proportion to the reduction in weight). This will be very clear from the raw measurements. Normalising the data, however, might suggest that there has been very little change in the load because the lower loads are divided by the lower body mass. The decision to normalise (and how) has to be made in the context of the clinical questions being asked.

The result of many normalisation schemes can be numbers that are unfamiliar to clinicians (Sutherland 1996). As non-dimensional normalisation becomes more widely applied in gait analysis, it may be that gait analysts develop a sense for whether a non-dimensional walking speed of 0.4 is fast or slow, but it is unlikely and unreasonable to expect that non-specialist clinicians will adopt this new approach. Sutherland suggested that dimensional units should be quoted as well as the non-dimensional equivalents but this in itself requires non-specialist to have a feel for the normal size of measurements. This may be reasonable for simple measures such as walking speed or stride length but is less so for more complex measurements such as hip abductor moment for example. An alternative is to express non-dimensional measurements as a percentage of the corresponding average measurement for the healthy population. Walking speed of 69% of average or peak hip abductor moment of 56% of average is quite understandable to most people. This is also analogous to the common practice of comparing gait traces from individual patients against normative reference data.

The effect of walking speed on data
Gait data are also affected by the speed at which a person walks. Effects of speed are not always obvious as all curves are time normalised to fit the gait graphs. Information about relative timing of features and the magnitude of the gait data are preserved by such scaling but the gradient of curves may be misleading. A slow walker may have difficulty moving into flexion or extension, for example, but when this is time normalised the gradient may appear normal. If angular or muscle lengthening velocities are considered to be clinically important, then they should be calculated and plotted rather than estimated from time-normalised plots of the respective angles or lengths. It is also important to remember that slower walkers spend a greater proportion of the gait cycle in both single and double support phases.

The definitive work of Schwartz et al. (2008) has established how gait data vary with the speed for children aged 4 to 17, and it is generally assumed that there will be similar effects for other age groups. Walking speed affects both the relative proportions of the different phases of gait within the gait cycle (e.g. stance phase as a percentage of the gait cycle decreases with walking speed) and all gait parameters and variables. Figure 2.17 illustrates joint angles measured at five different walking speeds. Some of the differences that occur naturally at low walking speeds such as reduced knee flexion in swing or reduced plantarflexion at toe off are assumed to be indicative of specific impairments

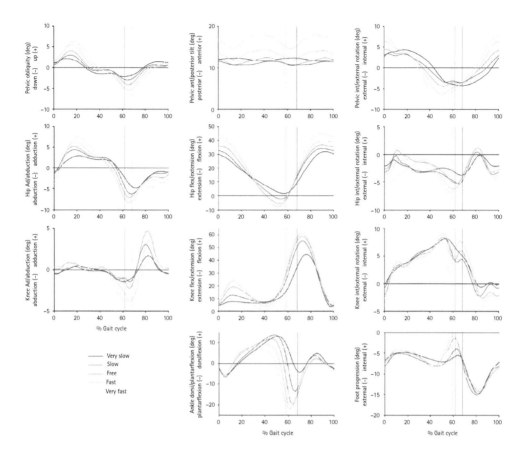

Figure 2.17 Variability of joint angles with walking speed in children aged 4 to 17 (Figure from Schwartz et al. 2008 with permission).

when observed in patients who often, of course, do walk slowly. Variability with speed is generally even greater for kinetic than kinematic data.

Whilst the work of Schwartz et al. has alerted the clinical community to this issue, there is little consensus on how it should be addressed in clinical interpretation. Most clinical services still present normative reference data collected at self-selected walking speed. There is an argument that a comparison with speed matched reference data would be more appropriate, but the details of how this should be done have not yet been described. No software capable of plotting data in this way is yet commercially available, and there has been no serious exploration of any potential disadvantages of this approach. For the foreseeable future, plotting reference data without matching for speed is likely to remain standard practice, but diligent analysts will make frequent reference to the study of Schwartz et al. when interpreting clinical results.

References

Alexander RM, Jayes AS. A dynamic similarity hypothesis for the gait of quadruped mammals. *J Zool Lond,* 1983, 201:135–152.

Baker R. Pelvic angles: a mathematically rigorous definition which is consistent with a conventional clinical understanding of the terms. *Gait Posture,* 2001, 13:1–6.

Baker R. Globographic visualisation of three dimensional joint angles. *J Biomech,* 2011, 44:1885–1891. DOI: 10.1016/j.jbiomech.2011.04.031

Dempster W. *Space requirements of the seated operator,* WADC Technical Report: 55–159. OH, Wright-Patterson Airforce Base, 1956.

Doorenbosch CA, Harlaar J, Veeger DH. The globe system: an unambiguous description of shoulder positions in daily life movements. *J Rehabil ResDev,* 2003, 40:147–155.

Hof A. Scaling gait data to body size. *Gait Posture,* 1996, 4:222–223.

Pearl M, Harris SL, Lippitt SB, Sidles JA, Harryman DTH, Matsen FA. A system for describing the positions of the humerus relative to the thorax and its use in the presentations of several functionally important arm positions. *J Shoulder Elbow Surg,* 1992, 1:113–118. DOI: 10.1016/S1058-2746(09)80129-8

Perry J. *Gait Analysis.* Thorofare, NJ, SLACK, 1992.

Schache AG, Baker R. On the expression of joint moments during gait. *Gait Posture,* 2007, 25:440–452.

Schache AG, Baker R, Vaughan CL. Differences in lower limb transverse plane joint moments during gait when expressed in two alternative reference frames. *J Biomech,* 2007, 40:9–19.

Schwartz MH, Koop SE, Bourke JL, Baker R. A nondimensional normalization scheme for oxygen utilization data. *Gait Posture,* 2006, 24:14–22.

Schwartz MH, Rozumalski A, Trost JP. The effect of walking speed on the gait of typically developing children. *J Biomech,* 2008, 41:1639–1650. DOI: 10.1016/j.jbiomech.2008.03.015

Strasser H. *Lehrbuch der Muskel und Gelenkmechanik.* Berlin, Springer, 1917.

Sutherland D. Dimensionless gait measurements and gait maturity. *Gait Posture,* 1996, 4:209–211.

Vaughan CL, Langerak NG, O'Malley MJ. Neuromaturation of human locomotion revealed by non-dimensional scaling. *Exp Brain Res,* 2003, 153:123–127.

Wu G, Cavanagh PR. ISB recommendations for standardization in the reporting of kinematic data. *J Biomech,* 1995, 28:1257–1261.

Wu G, Siegler S, Allard P, et al. ISB recommendation on definitions of joint coordinate system of various joints for the reporting of human joint motion – Part I: ankle, hip, and spine. International Society of Biomechanics. *J Biomech,* 2002, 35:543–548.

Zajac FE, Gordon ME. Determining muscle's force and action in multi-articular movement. *Exerc Sport Sci Rev,* 1989, 17:187–230.

Chapter 3
The conventional gait model

A biomechanical model allows us to reduce all the complexity of the human anatomy and the movements that occur during walking to something that is simple enough to understand. This is achieved by describing the complex shapes of the different bones as a manageable number of simple geometrical shapes. One particular model of the lower limbs has been far more widely accepted in clinical gait analysis than any other and is referred to here as the conventional gait model (CGM). Most system manufacturers implement some version of the model. For a variety of historical reasons, it is also known as the Newington, Davis, Gage, (Davis et al. 1991; Ounpuu et al. 1991, 1996), Helen Hayes or Kadaba (Kadaba et al. 1989, 1990) model. It is also sometimes referred to through manufacturer specific implementations such as Vicon's clinical manager (VCM) or plug-in gait (PiG).

The model was developed over 20 years ago when technology was considerably less advanced than it is now and consequently has significant limitations. Clinical governance provisions, however, dictate that only well-validated and well-understood models are suitable for processing patient data. Formal explicit validation of the CGM, as reported in the literature, is not strong, but it is stronger than that presented for any other model. Indeed the principal validation of other models has often been through comparison to the output of the CGM (Collins et al. 2009). There is substantial implicit validation of the CGM through the considerable number of research projects that have been based on its use. It is also by far the most widely used model for clinical gait analysis, and there are many more people within the clinical community who have a detailed understanding of its strengths and limitations than for any other model. Whilst other models have been proposed, there is, as yet, no convincing evidence that alternatives are any better. Alternative models are discussed in Chapter 4, but it is strongly recommended that, until an evidence base is developed to establish the superiority of any of these alternatives, the CGM should remain the model of choice for contemporary clinical gait analysis.

The CGM divides the body into seven segments (the pelvis and two femurs, tibias and feet). These segments are linked by joints that are all assumed to be ball and socket joints (three degrees of freedom). The position of each joint is defined within its proximal segment and used to define its distal segment. For example, the hip joint location is defined within the pelvis and then used to define the femur segment. The model is thus hierarchical from the pelvis down to the feet. If any segment cannot be defined, because of missing markers, for example, then none of the segments distal to this can be defined either.

The segments are defined from the measured positions of markers (how measurement systems calculate these positions is described in Chapter 15). Whilst the concept of segment coordinate systems (as introduced in Chapter 2) helps describe the precise definition of joint angles, most of the features of the CGM can be adequately appreciated if each segment is conceived of as a triangle. Any triangle is formed by a line and a point (the line itself is, of course, defined by two points) and lies in a specific plane. For the CGM, the line is the principal axis of the segment and the triangle lies in one of its anatomical planes. The position of the line tells us how the segment is aligned and the point allows us to measure how much rotation there is about that axis. To place markers accurately for the CGM, it is important to be able to imagine where these points, lines and triangles are within the body. The basics of the model are described in two sections: how the triangles are defined for each segment and how markers should be placed to allow the position of these segments to be calculated. Over time, a number of variants of the CGM have been developed, and the more common of these are also described.

Anatomical definition of segment triangles
Until recently, there has been some ambiguity as to whether segments should be related to the physical anatomy (on the basis of landmarks) or functional anatomy (the axes about which movement occurs at various joints). Widespread use of medical imaging is now placing increasing emphasis on defining segments in relation to the physical anatomy, and this is the primary approach that is adopted in this book.

Femur (Figure 3.1)
The long bones are the easiest to visualise. The primary axis is that between the proximal and distal joint centres. Thus for the femur, it is the line between the hip joint centre and the knee joint centre. If we know which direction this line is pointing in, then we know which direction the segment is pointing in and we can measure hip flexion and adduction. The point is the lateral epicondyle. If we know where this is in relation to the primary axis, then we know how much internal rotation there is. Together the line and the point create the triangle for the femur, which fully specifies its position and orientation.

Tibia (Figure 3.1)
The tibia is represented in the same way as the femur. The line is that between the proximal and distal joints, the knee joint centre and the ankle joint centre. The point is the lateral malleolus. Together these form the tibia triangle that specifies its position and orientation. The knee joint centre actually lies within the femur, and it is outside the

tibia This is not a conceptual problem in defining the tibia but does raise practical issues in how to place markers.

Pelvis (Figure 3.2)
The pelvis segment is based on the bony landmarks of the ilium rather than on the basis of the joint centres. The primary axis is that between the two anterior superior iliac spines (ASIS). This is chosen because, in a symmetrical pelvis, it is parallel to the line between the hip joint centres (the equivalent to the line between proximal and distal joints for the long bones). The point is the mid-point between the two posterior superior iliac spines. Together these form the pelvis triangle that specifies its position and orientation.

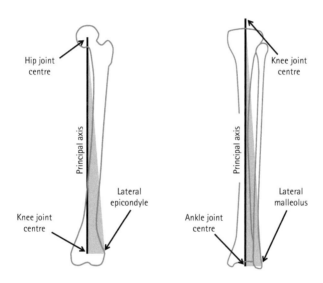

Figure 3.1 Anatomical definition of femur and tibia segments.

Figure 3.2 Anatomical definition of pelvis. ASIS, anterior superior iliac spine; PSIS, posterior superior iliac spine.

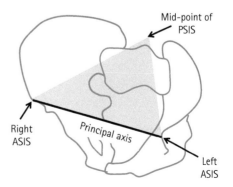

Foot (Figure 3.3)

The CGM was developed at a time when it was difficult to measure the position of more than two markers on the foot and as a consequence is only defined by a line (and not a triangle). In the undeformed foot, this line runs from the posterior aspect of the calcaneus through the hindfoot and along the second ray and is parallel to the plantar surface of the foot. This allows the alignment of this line to be specified but not the rotation around it (inversion).

Placing markers to define segment triangles

Although the segments defined above are anatomically meaningful, many of them are defined by points that are inside the body (such as joint centres) where it is impossible to place markers. The developers of the CGM therefore had to work out how to place markers in order to define these segments. Given the limitations of measurement technology at the time, they did so in a way that required a minimum number of markers, and it is this that resulted in the hierarchical approach described above.

Pelvis (Figure 3.4)

Placing markers to define the anatomical pelvis triangle is probably easier to understand than on the other segments because the triangle is defined directly by bony landmarks. These can generally be palpated through the skin and soft tissues. Markers have to be placed over both ASISs so that the marker centres define a line that runs parallel to the line between the actually bony landmarks. The pelvis point is an imaginary point that is half-way between the two posterior superior iliac spines (PSIS). Most modern users of the CGM place a marker over each of the PSIS. The mid-point between these and the line between the ASIS markers is used to form the pelvis marker triangle. If the markers are well placed, then this triangle and the anatomical femur

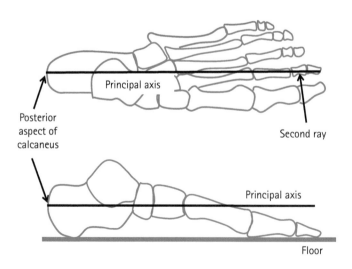

Figure 3.3 Anatomical definition of foot segment. The foot is only defined by its long axis and not by a triangle.

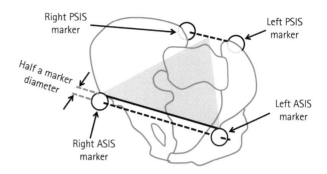

Figure 3.4 Placement of markers to define the pelvis segment. ASIS, anterior superior iliac spine; PSIS, posterior superior iliac spine.

triangle will lie in the same plane. This process is reasonably straightforward for lean people. For others the section later in this chapter on *Detailed guidance on pelvic marker placement (page 37)* should be consulted.

The anatomical triangle is posterior to the marker triangle by half the marker diameter. This is important to know in order for the position of the hip joint centre to be estimated in the next stage of the process, and the marker diameter thus has to be entered into the software. The mid-point of the PSIS markers is also behind that of the PSIS landmarks but because the point only defines the amount that the triangle is rotated about the line this is unimportant.

When the CGM was first developed, a single wand marker was used over the sacrum because measurement systems then in use often only had three cameras and could not detect skin-mounted markers. The marker triangle was then defined by this point and the line between the two ASIS markers. Today, virtually any modern system is able to detect two skin-mounted markers on the lower back, and such wand markers are now obsolete.

Femur (Figure 3.5)
How markers are placed on the femur to define the anatomical segment is a little more complex. The point that defines the femur triangle is the lateral epicondyle and one marker should be placed directly over this. The line, however, is between the hip and knee joint centres and is clearly not possible to place markers directly on either of these. The hip centre, however, links the pelvis and femur and can be considered as fixed in relation to both. If we know where the pelvis is then we can estimate where the hip joint centre is and use this as the second marker for the femur. Using data from radiographic studies of healthy adults (Davis et al. 1991), we can estimate how far out, back and down the hip joint is from the centre of the ASIS to ASIS line. The distances posterior, lateral and distal are calculated on the basis of leg length and ASIS to ASIS distance. Leg length must therefore be input to the software.

The next stage of defining the femur segment triangle requires us to know the plane in which it lies. That plane is defined by the hip joint centre and femoral condyle, which

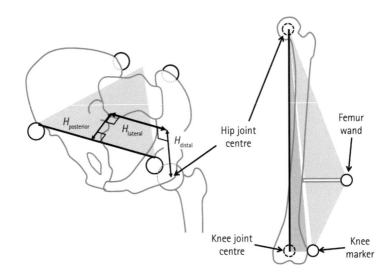

Figure 3.5 Placing markers to define the femur segment. $H_{posterior}$, $H_{lateral}$ and H_{distal} are the hip joint centre coordinates within the pelvic segment.

we already know, and the knee joint centre, which we do not know. We thus have to place a lateral femur wand marker in such a way that the triangle defined by it and the two other known points lies in the same plane as the anatomical femur triangle. This is one of the most challenging aspects of marker placement for the CGM and is described later in this chapter in the section, *Detailed guidance on determining the coronal plane of the femur* (page 39).

Once this plane has been defined, then the knee joint centre is defined as being half the knee width from the base-plate of the lateral epicondyle marker in the plane defined by the thigh markers. (The precise direction in which this distance is measured is chosen so that the line from the knee joint centre to the lateral epicondyle marker is perpendicular to the line between hip and knee joint centre.) Clearly this requires the knee width to be entered into the software. It also assumes that the knee marker is of the same diameter as the ASIS markers.

In recent years, there has been a tendency to replace the femur wand with a skin marker on the lateral thigh (this is even recommended in the PiG user manual). This creates a very narrow triangle, which means that small errors in placing either the knee or femur wand marker or small movements of the soft tissues will lead to large differences in the plane in which the femur marker triangle lies and hence to errors in measuring rotation about the line from hip to knee joint centre. Use of wand markers at the femur is thus essential. These may be subject to some wobble but using wands with firm bases securely taped to the thigh can generally reduce this to a minimum.

As suggested above, it is the position of the spherical marker that is detected by the measurement system and therefore the marker centre that must be in the correct plane. The exact position of the base-plate or the angles of the wand is unimportant, other than that the position of these will dictate where the marker centre ends up. Wand markers with a small ball and socket joint at the base of the wand are available which allow for easy adjustment of the alignment of wands. The soft tissues of the thigh move relative to the femur. Positioning this marker at about three-fourths of the distance from the hip to knee centre appears to be the best location for the femur wand (Lamoreux 1991; Schache et al. 2008).

Tibia (*Figure 3.6*)

The originators of the CGM chose to treat the tibia in essentially the same way as the femur. One marker is placed over the lateral malleolus. The knee links the femur and tibia and so the knee joint centre already defined for the femur is used for the tibia as well. A tibial wand marker is then used to define the plane of the femur segment triangle. The use of a wand marker is important for exactly the same reasons as for the femur. There is less soft tissue over the distal tibia than the proximal tibia so a position about two-thirds of the length from knee to ankle is optimal.

The ankle joint centre is then assumed to be half the ankle width in from the base-plate of the lateral malleolus marker in this plane in such a way that the line from the ankle joint centre to lateral malleolus is perpendicular to that to the knee joint centre. Again, it is assumed that the lateral malleolus marker is of the same diameter as the ASIS markers.

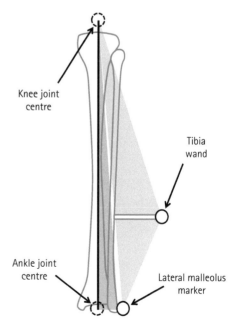

Figure 3.6 Placing markers to define the tibia.

Knee joint centre

Tibia wand

Ankle joint centre

Lateral malleolus marker

Foot (Figure 3.7)

A similar approach is adopted for the foot. The ankle joint centre links the tibia and foot so its position is taken from the tibia As there is only a line to define rather than a marker, then only one other marker is required, and this is the called the *foot* marker. The more distal this marker, the less sensitive the joint angles will be to a fixed error in marker placement and many centres choose a distal placement (on the metatarsals) when it may be referred to as a *toe* marker. If there is any foot deformity, however, this may not give an accurate indication of the alignment of the hindfoot, and if there is foot instability then movement of the joints within the foot might lead to erroneous measures of ankle dorsiflexion Most clinical services thus use a more proximal placement typically at about the level of the tarsometatarsal (Lisfranc) joints.

It can be seen from Figure 3.7 that at this level the long axis of the foot actually passes through the joint between the 2nd and 3rd proximal metatarsal heads, and so this is where the marker should be placed. As the ankle joint centre is generally medial to the long axis of the foot, however, the line from the ankle joint centre to the foot marker is generally at an angle to the long axis of the foot. This angle will be reasonably constant in standing and in walking; so a static calibration test is conducted to measure the offset and then this is used as a correction factor for walking trials. In order to calculate these angles, a heel marker is placed on the posterior aspect of the calcaneus such that the line from it to the foot marker lies along the long axis of the foot in the transverse plane. A similar issue exists in the sagittal plane, requiring the calculation of a plantarflexion offset during the static calibration test. The heel marker thus has to be placed in the same height above the plantar surface of the foot as the foot marker. Some software allows the

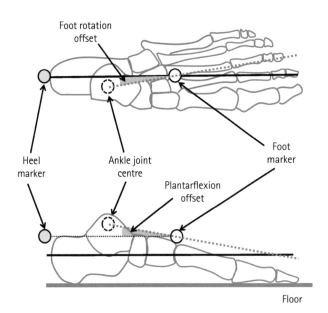

Figure 3.7 Placing markers to define the foot segment.

foot to be specified as flat in which case the plantarflexion offset will be calculated on the basis of the true horizontal rather than the relative heights of the two markers. This option should only be used if the person is standing with their full foot on the ground during the static calibration trail.

Detailed guidance on pelvic marker placement

The description of pelvic marker placement described in the section above works well in leaner young people. The pelvic landmarks can be easily palpated, markers can be placed while palpating the landmarks without displacing the soft tissues and the equations that estimate the hip joint centres do not require modification. Many people attending gait analysis, however, are more challenging. Among the young, the primary challenge comes from excess soft tissue around the pelvis. In the elderly, this can be exacerbated if the skin is of poor quality and the soft tissues sag. The key concept for placing pelvic markers in such people is to focus on the underlying principles of marker placement and adapt the technique accordingly.

The most important principle is that the markers must lie in the transverse plane of the pelvis (see Figure 3.8). This is defined as the plane containing the two ASIS landmarks

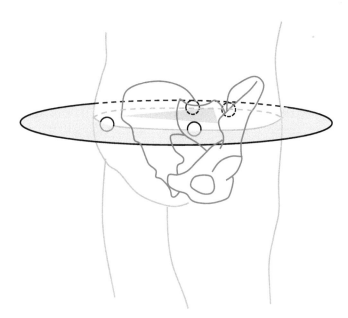

Figure 3.8 Visualising the extended transverse plane of the pelvis and placing markers over the landmarks where this intersects with the skin. The anterior superior iliac spine (ASIS) markers should be the same distance apart as the underlying landmarks. (Note that this plane is usually more anteriorly tilted than it appears in this figure.)

and the mid-point of the PSIS landmarks. The most important factor determining accurate marker placement is the analyst's ability to visualise where this plane lies. It should be stating the obvious that this is impossible without palpating the relevant landmarks. Thus, however deep the soft tissues, and even if this causes some discomfort to the patient, it is essential to palpate the landmarks. (Learning to do this without causing embarrassment is also an important skill for gait analysts to learn.) This must be done with the person standing. If markers are placed in other positions, particularly in lying, then the soft tissues will move when the person stands up and the markers will move with respect to the bony landmarks.

Once this plane has been visualised, the next requirement is that all four markers are placed on the line where this plane passes through the skin. The second requirement is that the ASIS markers are placed symmetrically. Remember that the line between these two markers defines the direction of the primary axis of the pelvis (mediolateral axis). If one is placed further forwards than the other, then this axis will not be properly defined. It is also important to remember that the position of the left and right hip joints is specified in relation to the point half-way between the ASIS markers; so if these markers are not placed symmetrically then the hip joint centres will not be symmetric either. The PSIS markers only define how the pelvic transverse plane is tilted about this axis, and the focus should be on their relative height with respect to the ASIS (although placing them symmetrically will still be good practice).

If the ASIS markers are separated from the ASIS landmarks by a thickness of soft tissue, then this needs correcting for in the equations that estimate hip joint position. In the most commonly used implementations, this is specified by the *ASIS to greater trochanter* distance. This is the distance between the base-plate of the ASIS marker and the greater trochanter (see Figure 3.9) in the horizontal direction. If this measure is the input to the software, then this will be used to estimate how far the hip joint centre is posterior to the ASIS marker; if not a regression equation will be used without making any allowance for soft tissues over the ASIS. It should be noted that because of femoral anteversion, the greater trochanter is generally a little posterior to the hip joint centre, and this measure will generally lead to the hip being a little too posterior relative to the pelvis. Correcting for this depends on both the degree of anteversion and the degree of internal hip rotation that the person is standing in when the measurement is made, and this error is generally tolerated (although simple geometrical estimates suggest this could lead to an error of up to 3cm in an adult with 45° of femoral anteversion). As with the placement of markers, this measurement should be made in standing. Measurements made in lying will be misleading if there is movement of the soft tissues when the person stands.

The lateral position of the hip joint centre is estimated on the basis of the *ASIS to ASIS distance*. By default, this will be calculated by the software from the measured position of the left and right ASIS markers during the static trial. In the presence of significant soft tissue, it may be difficult to guarantee that the markers are the same distance apart as the landmarks. In this case, the distance between the landmarks can be measured directly (based on palpation), and if this is entered in the software it will be used

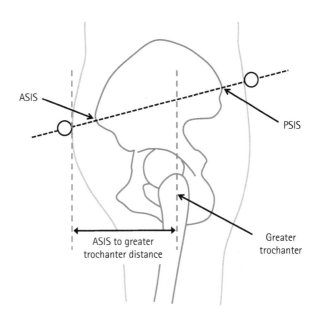

Figure 3.9 Use of ASIS to greater trochanter distance to estimate the position of the hip in the posterior direction. Note that in the figure, this will overestimate the distance by which the hip joint centre is posterior to the ASIS markers, which is one of the weaknesses of this implementation of the CGM. ASIS, anterior superior iliac spine; PSIS, posterior superior iliac spine.

instead. As this is a measurement of the bony anatomy, there is less of a problem in making this measurement in supine lying but it is still best practice to make it in standing.

Detailed guidance on determining the coronal plane of femur

As described above, the femur wand marker needs to be placed in such a way that it and the hip joint and knee marker lie in the coronal plane of the femur, which is defined as that containing the hip and knee joint centres and the lateral femoral epicondyle. This is extremely difficult to do in practice, which has led to a number of alternative procedures. None is entirely satisfactory, but most analysts will adopt one and learn to apply it to the best of their ability rather than trying to master all of them.

Direct femur wand alignment

The most direct method is simply to try to place the femur wand marker in the correct place to define the coronal plane of the femur. This is helped significantly using femur wands that have some degree of adjustability at the base. One manufacturer provides a small metal ball and socket joint between wand and base that can be adjusted and then fixed with a locking thread. Another manufacturer uses a plastic ball and socket where friction is sufficient to hold the position to which the wand is adjusted. With either device, the base can be fixed to the skin in approximately the correct position, and then fine adjustments can be made with the ball and socket joint.

Perhaps the best way to align the femur wand marker directly is to position the person so that the coronal plane of the hip is aligned with the global coronal plane during marker placement. In this position, the thigh marker should be adjusted so that it is in line with the knee marker and hip joint centre when viewed from the side. Whilst conceptually relatively straightforward, there are several practical difficulties with this approach.

The first difficulty is in positioning the person. It is best to have the person stand symmetrically with the pelvic coronal plane aligned with that of the global coronal plane. The femurs should then be aligned so that the line from the medial to lateral epicondyles lies in the global coronal plane as well. This can be done by asking the person to take their weight off one foot and then internally or externally rotating that limb to get the correct alignment. Once weight is placed back on the limb, it tends to hold it in reasonable alignment while the process is repeated for the other limb. Whilst the primary definition of the segment is anatomical, in most people the functional knee joint axis is very close to parallel to the transepicondylar axis. This can be used to check positioning. If the person performs a series of shallow squats in this position (with the help of a standing frame if necessary), then the knees should move directly backwards and forwards in the global sagittal plane.

The next difficulty is that in order to avoid parallax effects, the analyst should stand well back to give a true side view of the person. They are then however too far away to reach the thigh wands, and accurate alignment requires the analyst alternating adjustments to the thigh wands with stepping back to check that alignment. An alternative is to place a mirror parallel to the global sagittal plane a couple of metres lateral of the person on the side of the thigh marker to be adjusted. The analyst can then make the adjustment from the *other side* of the person looking past the thigh at the reflected image in the mirror. In this way, the alignment can be checked continuously whilst performing the adjustment.

The final difficulty is in estimating the hip joint centre. A reasonable compromise is to assume that the hip joint centre lies under the greater trochanter, and some people find it useful to place a marker over it. (It is preferable to place this marker on the skin but because it is only ever used as part of the alignment process it is less of an issue if it is placed on clothing than for other markers.) The same issue arises as with the *ASIS to greater trochanter* distance: particularly with people with marked femoral anteversion, the greater trochanter will generally lie a little anterior to the greater trochanter. As with that measure, this error is generally just accepted.

Use of a knee alignment device
An alternative to femur wand alignment is to accept that the thigh wand is not perfectly aligned but to calculate a correction factor to compensate for this. A static test is required from which the correction factor is calculated. The most common version of this uses a knee alignment device (KAD). This is a spring-loaded metal jig, which clamps on the medial and lateral epicondyles of the knee joint such that the line between the centres of the two clamp pads is parallel to the knee joint axis while the patient is standing. The KAD incorporates three markers that allow the position of the knee joint centre and the lateral knee marker (which cannot be placed until the KAD is removed) and the direction of this axis to be calculated. During the standing test, the

software can work out where the coronal plane of the femur is (i.e. that containing the hip and knee joint centres and the knee joint axis) and calculate the angle that the plane containing the hip and knee joint centres and the thigh marker makes with this. Once the KAD is removed, the lateral knee marker is placed and whenever data are processed subsequently, the correction factor is applied to correct for the actual alignments of the thigh marker.

This technique avoids any need to align the femur in any particular way, to be able to avoid parallax in viewing the femur segment or with estimating where the position of the hip joint centre is (the software will use the same algorithms to do this as are used to determine the position of the hip joint centre during walking). It is solely dependent, however, on how accurately the analyst can align the KAD. This can be considerably more difficult than the instructions suggested above. The medial and lateral knee pads are fixed and parallel and do not always sit easily on the contours of the epicondyles as required. Both epicondyles are quite broad landmarks, and a certain amount of judgement is required to define the precise alignment required. Many people recommend visualising the hinge axis of the knee joint by performing shallow squats, but this is extremely difficult to do accurately. The KAD becomes even more unstable with knee movement, so this can be counter-productive. Care is also needed to ensure that the lateral knee marker is placed in the correct position after the KAD is removed (the centre of this marker should lie over the same point on the lateral epicondyle that the lateral KAD pad was centred on).

There are particular issues if the person stands with the knee in a markedly different degree of flexion to that during walking. This most often occurs when a patient stands in full extension or hyperextension but walks predominantly in flexion. Skin movement over the knee means that the lateral epicondyle marker may be in a different position relative to the femur during standing and walking, and this will introduce an artefact into the data. Arranging for the person to stand with a knee flexion similar to that adopted during the stance phase of gait is one way to overcome this (note that this requires the analyst to have briefly observed how the person is walking before he or she starts placing markers).

Use of a medial epicondyle marker
A variant on the KAD that avoids some of the problems is to apply lateral and medial epicondyle markers for the static trial. In theory, the software can calculate exactly the same information provided by the KAD on the basis of just these two markers, and there are none of the problems associated with how the KAD sits on the knee or with replacing the knee marker in the same position as the lateral KAD pad. The medial epicondyle marker is best removed after the static test as it commonly gets knocked off by the other knee in gait during walking anyway. Occasionally, patients will stand with the knees together, preventing the placement of medial epicondyle markers. This can generally be worked around by placing a small pillow or bolster between the thighs to separate the knees. Care should be taken to ensure that this does not affect the position of the thigh wands. Unfortunately few manufacturers have made this option available in their software.

Detailed guidance on determining the coronal plane of the tibia

Direct tibial wand alignment
Similar issues exist for the tibia and similar solutions are possible. Thus doing everything possible to align the tibial wand correctly is one option. In doing this, it is necessary to remember that the tibia coronal plane is that containing the knee and ankle joint centres and the lateral malleolus. Unless tibial torsion is zero, which is very rare, it is not possible to align the coronal plane of the tibia with the global coronal plane at the same time as the femur. Most analysts using this technique will thus attempt to place the tibial wands by eye without aligning the tibia. In this they are trying to place the tibial marker in the same plane as that containing the medial and lateral malleoli and the knee joint centre. This can generally be assessed reasonably well looking down on the tibia from the front and may well be helped by placing an extra marker on the medial malleolus simply to guide tibial wand placement during the static trial. In doing this, it should be remembered that the proximal point defining the tibial coronal plane is the knee joint centre and not the lateral epicondyle marker.

Use of a medial malleolar marker
Rather than just using the medial malleolar marker to visualise the ankle joint axis, it is, of course, possible to use it to define the ankle joint axis and use this as a basis for working out a correction factor for tibial wand misalignment. This is a commonly available option and is probably the most sensible for routine clinical use. Whilst they look vulnerable, small medial malleolar markers are often not knocked off during walking and can thus be left on. Whilst not contributing to the gait data captured during walking, they can be useful if there is any reason to repeat the static calibration.

Using a clinical measure of tibial torsion
Early users of the KAD made use of a clinical measure of tibial torsion to determine a correction factor for tibial alignment. If tibial torsion is the angle between the knee joint axis and the ankle joint axis in the transverse plane, then it is also the angle between the coronal plane of the femur and that of the tibia in standing. Thus if the KAD has been used to determine the coronal plane of the femur, tibial torsion can be used to determine the coronal plane of the tibia and thus as a basis to calculate the angle by which the tibial wand lies out of this plane.

The main limitation of this technique is the accuracy with which it is possible to measure tibial torsion, which is one of the more difficult anthropometric parameters to measure. Indeed one of the advantages of the other two methods is that they can be used to generate a value for tibial torsion that can be compared with the clinical measure for quality assurance purposes.

Detailed guidance on foot marker placement in the presence of foot pathology
One of the most significant limitations of the CGM is that it regards the foot as the only one segment that is defined by a single axis. This is quite reasonable for the healthy foot

in which the bones are well aligned, and that single axis is reasonably well defined. In the deformed foot, however, the long axis of the forefoot may be pointing in quite a different direction to that of the hindfoot (see Figure 3.10). Using a distal toe marker will define a composite long axis which does not represent either. It is for this reason that a more proximal placement is used (over the joint of the 2nd and 3rd proximal metatarsal heads). The long axis thus defined reflects the long axis of the hindfoot. This has parallels in the physical assessment of dorsiflexion in which, in the presence of foot deformities, it is the plantar surface of the hindfoot which is taken as the reference and not that of the whole foot. It should be noted that in a planus foot (see Figure 3.10), this may still result in the foot marker being a little lateral, and the heel marker may need to be placed slightly lateral of the most posterior aspect of the heel to correct for this. In a cavus foot, an opposite effect may occur requiring a slightly more medial placement.

Use of the floor

Placing the heel marker at the correct height accurately is difficult and a potential source of error. If the foot can be placed flat on the floor, then it is more reliable to assume that the long axis of the hindfoot is parallel to the floor during standing than that the heel marker has been placed at the correct height. Most softwares allow the operator to flag that this is the case and calculate the sagittal plane offset on this assumption. The heel marker still has to be placed in the correct position in the transverse plane.

Adapting the conventional gait model for shoe, orthoses and prostheses

Clearly, the forefoot and heel markers will have to be placed on shoes if worn. The same basic principles are used for palpating the markers. The phalanges of the second ray can often be palpated through the shoe, but if not, aligning markers with the midline of the forefoot section of the shoe may be more appropriate. It is virtually impossible to adjust markers for foot deformities within shoes. This may need to be taken into account when reporting differences in foot progression and ankle internal rotation when comparing shod and barefoot conditions. The other issue is that of the pitch of the shoe, which is

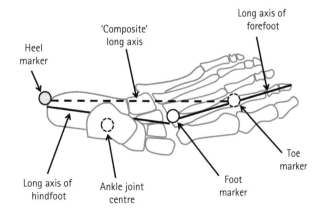

Figure 3.10 A foot with a planus deformity.

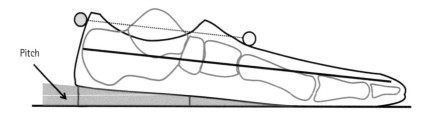

Figure 3.11 Placement of heel and forefoot markers for a pitched shoe.

the angle that the inside of the sole makes with the ground (see Figure 3.11). If the pitch is appreciable then the plantar surface and hence the long axis of the foot will be pitched forwards. The line between the forefoot and heel marker during the static should then be parallel to the inside of the shoe rather than the ground (see Figure 3.11), and in this case the foot flat option should not be selected. (Some software allows the pitch angle to be measured and entered into the software allowing the foot flat option to be selected even in shoes.)

If orthoses are worn then the markers will often have to be placed on these rather than on the skin. The same alignment principles are required, with the marker centres being placed on the appropriate joint axes or in the correct planes. Orthoses may not be symmetrical around the knee and ankle joints, and in this case the knee width entered into the software should be twice the distance from the base-plate of the lateral marker to the joint centre rather than the actual knee width. The same applies for placing markers on prostheses. These may not have equivalents to the bony landmarks used to place skin markers. Sensible assumptions are generally possible if the general principles outlined above have been understood.

Practical guidelines for use of conventional gait model

Anthropometric measures
Most measurements should be made in lying before data capture and are best incorporated into the physical examination.

ASIS to ASIS distance   The mediolateral distance between the left and right ASIS measured with either callipers or a tape measure. If a tape measure is being used, then care is required to measure the straight line distance between the markers and not that around any abdominal soft tissues. Some software can calculate this from the distance between the left and right ASIS markers during the static calibration if the value is omitted (this option should only be used if the analyst is confident that markers are the same distance apart as the underlying landmarks).

Leg length	The distance between the ASIS and the medial malleolus on the same side with the knee extended. In patients with knee flexion contractures, this should be measured as the sum of the distance from ASIS to medial epicondyle and from medial epicondyle to medial malleolus.
Knee width	The distance across the knee from the skin over the medial epicondyle to that over the lateral epicondyle. This can easily be made with an anthropometer. Minimal compression should be applied while measuring as the tissues are not compressed during walking.
Ankle width	The distance across the ankle from the skin over the medial malleolus to that over the lateral malleolus. This can easily be made with an anthropometer. Minimal compression should be applied while measuring as the tissues are not compressed during walking.
ASIS to trochanter distance	The distance in the posterior direction from the base-plate of the ASIS marker to the greater trochanter, which is taken as an estimate of how far the hip joint centre is posterior to the ASIS marker (Figure 3.9). This measurement should really be made in standing as soft tissues over the pelvis will be differently distributed in lying. Most software will calculate a default value for this value based on leg length and ASIS to ASIS distance. This should not be used if there is significant soft tissue over the pelvis.

Marker placement

Markers are placed to define either lines or planes. The only part of the marker that the gait analysis system can see is the retroreflective sphere and the only thing it measures is the position of the centre of that sphere (see Figure 3.12). It is, therefore, important when placing markers that the centre of that sphere is located accurately. If a line is being defined then the marker centre has to be placed on that line. If a plane is being defined then the marker centre needs to be placed in that plane. The position of the marker base-plate is only important to the extent to which it determines where the marker centre lies. Of course the lines and planes are imaginary so the key to good marker placement is being able to imagine where these lines and planes are. This in turn requires a clear understanding of the location of bony landmarks and how to palpate these accurately. Brief descriptions of these are given below, but readers are referred to van Sint Jan's excellent volume for further details (van Sint Jan 2007).

Markers should always be applied in standing. Markers placed during sitting or lying will move in relation to the bones as a consequence of soft tissue and skin movements as the patient stands. This will lead to erroneous definition of segments and thus of kinematics and kinetics. Some people may have difficulty standing unassisted for the time taken for marker placement and will require the use of a standing frame. This can

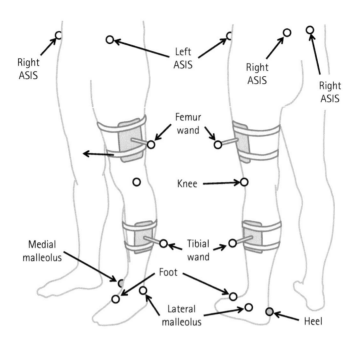

Figure 3.12 Markers required for the conventional gait model. Only markers on the left limb are illustrated for clarity. Markers with grey fill are only required for a static trial. ASIS, anterior superior iliac spine.

either be a conventional walking frame (preferably one without any wheels) or one built especially for the purpose that includes a small seat or perch. Most motion capture systems have sufficient cameras to see around such a frame but painting it a dark matt colour might help prevent extraneous reflections that can cause problems for some systems. Most people who can walk far enough to give a useful gait analysis will be able to stand with such assistance for the time taken to place markers (they can sit for rests if necessary). If standing is a particular problem, then applying tibial and foot markers in sitting may be reasonable but pelvis, thigh and knee markers should always be placed in standing. Whenever possible, the person should stand with heels on the ground with the knees in neutral extension (erring on the side of flexion is generally preferable to hyperextension).

Markers should always be attached directly to the skin and not on clothing. Markers on clothing, even it appears tight fitting or is well taped or strapped down, will tend to move with respect to the underlying bones. This will give rise to unreliable segment definition and hence erroneous kinematics and kinetics.

Lateral malleolus   This is placed over the lateral malleolus such that the centre of the marker lies on the line between the medial and lateral malleoli.

Medial malleolus | This marker is only required if it is to be used in for calculation of tibial rotation offsets during static calibration. It is placed over the medial malleolus such that the centre of the marker lies on the line between the lateral and medial malleoli.

Foot | This is placed over the joint between the proximal heads of the 2nd and 3rd metatarsals.

Heel | This marker is only required for calculating foot dorsiflexion and rotation offsets during the static calibration. It is placed on the posterior aspect of the heel such that the line between the centres of the foot and heel markers is parallel to the long axis of the hind foot. The heel marker should thus be the same distance above the plantar surface of the hind foot as the foot marker is. It should also be aligned in the transverse plane. In the healthy foot, the heel marker will generally be over the posterior aspect of the distal Achilles tendon. In the presence of foot deformities, it may need to be placed more medially (cavus feet) or laterally (planus feet).

Tibial wand | The base-plate is placed on the lateral aspect of the leg about a third of the way between ankle and knee. If direct wand alignment is being used, the centre of the marker should lie in the same plane as the medial and lateral malleoli and the knee joint centre. If the KAD or medial malleolar markers are used for calculating a tibial rotation offset, then the alignment of this marker is unimportant. In this case, it should be possible to place the base-plate such that the wands point anteriorly, which may reduce the likelihood of markers being knocked if the person uses walking aids.

Knee | This is placed over the lateral epicondyle such that the centre of the marker is on the line between the medial and lateral epicondyles. The iliotibial band can sometimes move anteriorly over the epicondyle with knee extension or hyperextension, leading to potential soft tissue artefact. This should be avoided by having the person stand with a neutral or mildly flexed knee. If the KAD is being used, then the knee marker cannot be placed until after the static calibration has been performed (and should be placed over the centre of the lateral knee pad of the KAD).

Femur wand | The base-plate is placed on the lateral aspect of the thigh about one-quarter of the distance from the knee to the hip. If direct wand alignment is being used, the centre of the marker should lie in the same plane as the medial and lateral epicondyles and the hip joint centre. If the KAD is used for calculating a femoral rotation offset, then the alignment of this marker is unimportant. In this case, it should be possible to place the base-plate such that the wands point anteriorly, which may reduce the likelihood of markers being knocked if the person uses walking aids.

ASIS	In people with minimal subcutaneous soft tissue, this marker is placed directly over the corresponding landmark. If there is significant soft tissue, then the marker should be placed such that its centre lies in the plane containing that two ASIS landmarks and the mid-point of the PSIS but still lies over the ASIS landmark in the pelvic coronal plane (i.e. the two ASIS markers should be the same distance apart as the ASIS landmarks).
PSIS	Placement of PSIS markers is analogous to that of the ASIS markers.
KAD	The KAD should be placed such that the lateral pad is centred over the centre of the lateral epicondyle and the medial pad is placed over the centre of the medial epicondyle. It is only its alignment in the transverse plane that is important (it does not matter if it is horizontal or not).

Conventional data capture

Data capture for the CGM requires the patient to stand still for a static trial (with the KADs in place if used) to allow the different offsets to be calculated. The patient should stand reasonably upright for this, and knee hyperextension should be avoided as this can displace knee markers anteriorly with respect to the bones. Calibration of plantarflexion offsets is more reliable if the plantar surface of the foot is on the ground and the foot flat assumptions can be used. This is possible for most patients but may require different calibration poses for the left and right limbs. It is worth understanding how the software works in order to achieve this (it may require intentionally not labelling markers on the other limb). For less stable walkers, a standing frame may be useful. Calibrations should not be performed seated as this can result in considerable soft tissue movement particularly under the pelvic markers.

Walking is generally straightforward. Most centres capture data at a self-selected walking speed. Standardised instructions such as 'walk at the speed you would normally choose to walk along a corridor' should be used. If collecting data for research purposes, then rigid protocols should be adhered to, but for general clinical purposes further instruction to speed up or slow down may be appropriate particularly with young children. Setting up the laboratory so that data can be captured in both directions will generally halve the overall time for data capture and may help avoid fatigue. It may also help in diagnosing faults in force plate set-up (see Chapter 11). Patients should generally be given a few 'practice' walks, allowing them to get used to walking in the laboratory environment before data capture starts (although this may not be wise for more marginal walkers who are only likely to be able to walk for a short time).

If kinetic data are required, then the analyst needs to ensure that one foot is entirely within the boundaries of a force plate and that neither the other foot nor any walking aid makes contact with the plate. In order to do this, the analyst must have a clear view of the force plates and clean contacts should be noted after each trial has been captured. Most patients have a reasonably consistent step length, and thus adjusting the starting point of the walk (in both an anterior–posterior and mediolateral direction) can help capture kinetics optimally. Having coloured markings on the floor to mark potential starting points can be very helpful (parallel lines about 20cm apart). Having these placed symmetrically to the force plates at both ends of the walkway should allow effective data capture whichever direction the patient is walking. Most services avoid drawing the patient's attention to where the force plates are in order that their gait pattern is not affected by the attempts to hit them. If particular difficulty is found in obtaining kinetics, however, then pointing out where the plates are might be sensible – kinetic data obtained through such targeting is likely to be more useful than no kinetic data at all.

Capturing data under different conditions such as with or without shoes or orthoses or with different walking aids takes additional time, and it is best to concentrate on a small number of these. Conditions requiring putting on and removing orthoses, shoes or clothing and replacing markers may also require repeat subject calibration and will clearly take longer than simply changing walking aids. Most clinicians will want to know about the inherent walking ability of the patient, which will generally be best assessed in bare feet with the minimum of aids required for reasonable walking. They will also generally be interested in how a patient walks with their usual combination of orthoses, shoes and walking aids. Concentrating on these two conditions is generally sufficient but others may be required at times.

Systems should be established to ensure that each session and trial has a unique identifier. Incorporating patient identifiers within this can make it easier to recognise data files but is obviously inappropriate if anonymisation of data is required. A log should be kept throughout data capture, recording details of different conditions, which force plate data are reliable and any other features of particular trials. This can be on paper but is much better if recorded on the computer along with the data.

References

Collins TD, Ghoussayni SN, Ewins DJ, Kent JA A six degrees-of-freedom marker set for gait analysis: repeatability and comparison with a modified Helen Hayes set. *Gait Posture,* 2009, 30:173–180. DOI: 10.1016/j.gaitpost.2009.04.004

Davis R, Ounpuu S, Tyburski D, Gage JR A gait analysis data collection and reduction technique. *Hum Mov Sci,* 1991, 10:575–587.

Kadaba MP, Ramakrishnan HK, Wootten ME, Gainey J, Gorton G, Cochran GV. Repeatability of kinematic, kinetic, and electromyographic data in normal adult gait. *J Orthop Res,* 1989, 7:849–860.

Kadaba MP, Ramakrishnan HK, Wootten ME. Measurement of lower extremity kinematics during level walking. *J Orthop Res,* 1990, 8:383–392.

Lamoreux L Errors in thigh axial rotation measurements using skin mounted markers. Proceedings of International Society of Biomechanics, Perth, Australia, 1991.

Ounpuu O, Davis R, Deluca P. Joint kinetics: methods, interpretation and treatment decision-making in children with cerebral palsy and myelomeningocele. *Gait Posture,* 1996, 4:62–78.

Ounpuu S, Gage J, Davis RB. Three-dimensional lower extremity joint kinetics in normal pediatric gait. *J Pediatr Orthop,* 1991, 11:341–349.

Schache AG, Baker R, Lamoreux LW. Influence of thigh cluster configuration on the estimation of hip axial rotation *Gait Posture,* 2008, 27:60–69.

van Sint Jan S. *Color atlas of skeletal landmark definitions: Guidelines for reproducible manual and virtual palpations.* London: Churchill Livingstone, 2007.

Chapter 4

Alternatives to the conventional gait model

Six degrees of freedom models

The most common alternative to the hierarchical conventional gait model (CGM) is a family of models probably best referred to as six degrees of freedom (6DoF) models. Variants include the Cleveland Clinic Markerset (which was implemented in the Motion Analysis Corporation's Orthotrak software) and the Calibrated Anatomical Systems Technique (CAST; Cappozzo et al. 1995). 6DoF techniques have become particularly popular as they are the basis of the Visual3D software from C-motion Inc. (Germantown, MD, USA). The variety of 6DoF models is even more bewildering than the variants of the CGM, and they are generally quite poorly documented in the academic literature. Despite widespread use, for example, there is no published description of the Cleveland Clinic Markerset. Two notable exceptions are the CAST technique and related implementations, which have been developed at the Istituti Ortopedici Rizzoli (IOR) in Bologna The developers refer to these as the plate-mounted protocol and the IOR model (Leardini et al. 2007).

The characteristic of these models is that they assume that each segment is independent of the others. Three joint angles still reflect the relative orientation of the different segments in space but do not assume that these occur about a fixed joint centre. It is therefore also possible to define three translations for each joint; hence the term *six* degrees of freedom. In order to measure this movement, it is necessary to place at least three markers on each segment, and these are referred to as a *cluster*. The earlier 6DoF models mounted these on rigid base plates (rigid clusters), which are strapped or taped to the femur or tibia Rigid clusters strapped over the sacrum to track the pelvis or to the feet have been proposed, but most modern models use clusters of skin-mounted markers for the pelvis and feet. Both the CAST (Cappozzo et al. 1995) and IOR models (Leardini et al. 2007) use multiple skin-mounted markers for the femur and tibia as well.

These markers (often referred to as *technical* or *tracking* markers) allow the definition of a technical coordinate system (Cappozzo et al. 2005). Whilst guidance is generally given on roughly where to place them, their exact positioning is unimportant because a calibration trial is used to establish the relationship between the technical coordinate system and an anatomical coordinate system based on the anatomical landmarks. The fundamental assumption of 6DoF models is that this relationship established during static standing calibration continues to be valid during walking (i.e. the cluster markers do not move with respect to the segments that they represent). The CAST technique originally proposed use of a pointer (two markers attached in known positions to a thin rod) to identify the landmarks during anatomical landmark calibration as a way of reducing the number of markers required during any single trial. Most modern systems are technically capable of measuring the position of large numbers of markers, and it is now almost universal to place additional calibration markers over the landmarks for the static trial (these can be left on during walking and this is useful if there is any reason why a repeat calibration might be required [Leardini et al. 2007]).

Comparison of anatomically defined segments
There is a general agreement that the anatomical definition of the pelvis and femur is essentially the same as outlined in Chapter 3 for the CGM. However, there is some variability across different models as to how the hip joint centre is calculated (Della Croce et al. 2005). The use of regression equations is common, but there is little consensus regarding which particular regression equations should be used. Functional calibration of the hip for 6DoF models has been reported (Collins et al. 2009).

The IOR model (Leardini et al. 2007) uses the anatomical segment definitions on which the CAST is based (Cappozzo et al. 1995), which differ from the CGM subtly for the tibia and quite markedly for the foot. The primary axis of the tibia does not go to the knee joint centre but to a point defined by the fibular head and tibial tuberosity in such a way that the two malleoli and the fibula head lie in the tibial coronal frame, and the tibial tuberosity and the mid-point of the malleoli lie in the tibia sagittal plane (see Figure 4.1).

In the CAST/IOR models the foot is defined quite differently to that of the CGM, with its definition not depending on the ankle joint centre at all. The posterior calcaneus marker in the middle of the upper ridge of the calcaneus' posterior surface and markers on the dorsal surface of the forefoot over the distal heads of the 1st and 5th metatarsals define the transverse plane of the foot. The sagittal plane is defined as being perpendicular to this and containing the posterior calcaneus marker and a calibration marker over the distal head of the 2nd metatarsal.

Comparison between technical marker sets
Because the static calibration defines the relationship between the technical cross-section and the anatomical cross-section for each individual placement, the exact locations of the technical markers are quite arbitrary at one level. Approximate positions are all that are required of any protocol. Most examples of the 6DoF approaches, however, use at least some markers for tracking *and* calibration. For example, most models use the

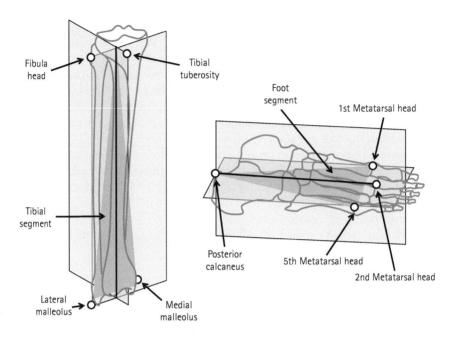

Figure 4.1 Anatomical segment definition for the tibia and foot in the calibrated anatomical systems technique (CAST) and Istituti Ortopedici Rizzoli (IOR) models. The metatarsal head markers are placed on the dorsal aspect of the relevant bones (Cappozzo et al. 1995).

ASIS and PSIS markers to both track and calibrate the pelvis. It is important that the analyst fully appreciates which markers have this shared purpose and need to be placed accurately and which are used only for tracking which do not.

Three broad approaches are adopted. The Cleveland Clinic Markerset uses rigid clusters of markers mounted on plates that are strapped to the femur and tibia sections (see Figure 4.2a). Given that the fundamental assumption of 6DoF modelling is that the tracking markers do not move relative to the underlying bones, it is essential that firm strapping or taping is used for this. This original Markerset used skin-mounted markers on the pelvis but others have proposed using rigid (Cappello et al. 1997; Benedetti et al. 1998) or skin marker (Seay et al. 2008) clusters here as well. The original description of CAST (Cappozzo et al. 1995) is largely conceptual and gives little guidance on placement of technical markers, but Figure 5 (page 176) of that paper implies the use of skin-mounted markers distributed over the mid-section of the segment. Later work from the same group (Cappozzo et al. 1997) suggested that placing the technical markers far apart would minimise the effect of a fixed magnitude of placement error or soft tissue artefact, but this can lead to placement of markers around the joint where considerable soft tissue artefact can be anticipated. The IOR model aims to reduce the number of markers required by using joint calibration and technical markers wherever possible, which

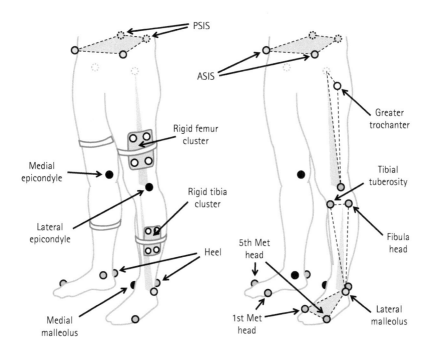

Figure 4.2 Modified Cleveland Clinic Markerset (left) and IOR model (right). White-filled markers are purely for tracking, grey-filled markers are both for tracking and for anatomical calibration, black-filled markers are for calibration only. Hip joint centres are estimated using regression equations. Grey shapes are anatomical segments whereas dotted grey lines link tracking markers. ASIS, anterior superior iliac spine; PSIS, posterior superior iliac spine.

has resulted in well-spaced markers on the segments. All three approaches use surface-mounted markers on the feet, although some groups with a special interest in the foot have used rigid clusters here as well (Benedetti et al. 1998; Nester et al. 2007).

Kinematic fitting

The most recent development in biomechanical modelling for gait analysis has been variously referred to as *global optimisation, inverse kinematics* and *kinematic fitting*. The last term is used in this book. These techniques have not yet been fully validated for clinical gait analysis but are likely to form the basis of future developments. Again the body is modelled as a number of rigid segments, but these are assumed to be linked at joints. Markers are then assumed to be located on specific segments. Clearly if the joints of the model are manipulated, the model will assume different poses and the markers on different segments will move relative to each other. In the fitting process, the model is manipulated so that all the model markers are as close as possible to the measured position of the real markers.

The fitting has two elements. *Model calibration* is the equivalent of anatomical calibration of a 6DoF model in which the dimensions of the segments and the locations of the markers are adjusted to fit the dimensions of the person being analysed and the locations at which the markers have been placed. In *tracking* the pose of the model is adjusted to give the best fit of the calibrated model to the measured positions of the markers throughout the trial. It is possible to combine both elements in one process (Charlton et al. 2004; Reinbolt et al. 2005) but more common for the two stages to be separated (Lu and O'Connor 1999).

Kinematic fitting has many advantages (see Figure 4.3). Perhaps the most important is that it provides a systematic approach to describing any biomechanical model (6DoF models can be seen as a special case). Joints can be modelled with different properties to match joint anatomy. The hip can be considered to move as a ball and socket joint with three rotational degrees of freedom, the ankle as a universal joint with two and the knee (over part of its range of motion) as a hinge with one. It is also possible to allow translational degrees of freedom or even more complex joints such as a knee joint, which translates as a function of joint angle (Yamaguchi and Zajac 1989). Most approaches so far assume that the markers are placed at fixed locations with respect to the different segments, but it is conceptually reasonably straightforward to model soft tissue artefact as a function of joint angles or statistically incorporate this into the fitting algorithm (Cappello et al. 2005). Tracking is usually performed on a frame-by-frame basis, but

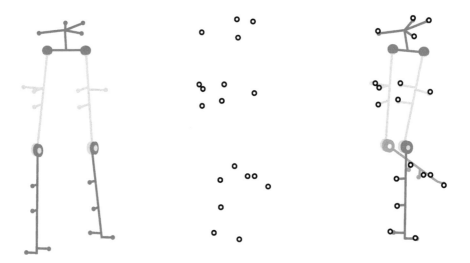

Figure 4.3 An example of kinematic fitting. A model is defined with five segments, each with a number of markers attached. The segments are linked to each other with joints of known properties (left). The measured positions of the markers are captured (centre). The joints are then manipulated to get the best match between the model markers and the measured markers (right).

various techniques are available to constrain joint angles to vary smoothly across frames, which effectively builds a filter into the fitting process. Kinematic fitting can also be adapted easily to incorporate functional calibration (see the next section, *Functional calibration*), to identify rotation axes and points from elementary joint motion.

There are further benefits if advanced processing techniques (see Chapter 6) are going to be used as the same model that has been used for kinematic fitting can be used both for muscle length modelling and for kinetic analysis. Given that the joint constraints are known, rigorous forward and inverse dynamic analyses can be performed without the need for corrections for joint translations (inherent in 6DoF models) or deformable segments (which are implicit in the segment definitions of the CGM) such as proposed by Kuo (1998). It is even possible to incorporate forward or inverse dynamic outputs into the tracking algorithms to ensure that the model matches the measured kinetics as well as the kinematics of movement (Thelen et al. 2003; Thelen and Anderson 2006). This approach is still at a developmental stage and has not yet been appropriately validated for clinical use.

Kinematic fitting gives more flexibility in the placement of markers. Markers for 6DoF models are optimal when placed furthest apart especially along the principal axis of the segment (Cappozzo et al. 1997). This requires markers to be placed close to the knee and hip which are prone to considerable soft tissue artefact (Lamoreux 1991; Schache et al. 2008; Tsai et al. 2009; Akbarshahi et al. 2010). Constraining movement to occur at joints between rigid segments results in more useful information being obtained from markers placed towards the middle of segments. It also allows information about the segments that are less prone to soft tissue artefact to assist in measuring the orientation of other segments those that are more prone (Lucchetti et al. 1998). Recent studies, for example, suggest soft tissue over specific locations on the tibia is minimal (Peters et al. 2009). Kinematic fitting allows optimal use of information from markers placed at those locations. It also allows information on tibial position to contribute to determining femur and even pelvic position, which are both more prone to soft tissue artefact.

Functional calibration

Functional calibration (Sommer 1980; Areblad 1990; van der Bogert et al. 1994) is often associated with kinematic fitting but can be incorporated into any biomechanical model. It involves determining some characteristics of the model, most often joint positions and axis orientations, on the basis of the movement data rather than the locations of landmarks. Therefore as the hip is a ball and socket joint, a marker on the femur will be expected to move on the surface of a sphere fixed in the pelvis with its centre at the hip joint centre. By analysing the movement data, it is possible to estimate the location of the hip joint centre without knowing anything specific about where the markers are positioned other than that they are on the two segments. The quality of functional calibration is determined by the extent to which the actual movement of the joint matches the movement assumed by the model (e.g. how closely the movement of a patient's knee can be represented by a hinge joint), the range of joint movement used for the calibration and the amount of soft tissue movement. It is possible to use data from the movement occurring during walking for functional calibration (Charlton et al. 2004), but there is not necessarily a suitable range of movement for this to be reliable.

Functional calibration of the hip appears to have most to offer the gait analyst. The joint cannot be palpated directly, and it is assumed that interindividual anatomical variability will lead to errors in estimates of its centre based on regression equations from those pelvic landmarks that can be palpated. Significant soft tissue over those landmarks may further reduce confidence in such estimates. Movement of the hip is assumed to closely approximate that of a ball and socket joint, which offers an excellent basis for functional calibration (Piazza et al. 2001). A number of different computational techniques are possible (Leardini et al. 1999; Schwartz and Rozumalski 2005; Chang and Pollard 2007a), which have been reviewed (Ehrig et al. 2006), and optimal calibration exercises have been specified (Camomilla et al. 2006). It is tempting to assume that a large range of motion is required, but this may not be the case if this increases soft tissue artefact. Some components of motion, such as internal and external rotation of the hip, may also give rise to large soft tissue artefact and may be best avoided.

Early studies suggested that such techniques gave better agreement than regression equations against radiological or ultrasound images (Leardini et al. 1999; Hicks and Richards 2005). Much of this apparent benefit, however, may be because of the particular choice of regression equations used. Recent work suggests that Harrington's MRI-based regression equations for hip joint centre (Harrington et al. 2007) perform at least as well as functional calibration for able-bodied adults (Sangeux et al. 2011) under tightly controlled research conditions and better than functional calibration in children with disability in a routine clinical service environment (Peters et al. 2012). It is also important to remember that some people seen routinely for gait analysis may have hip pathology that renders the ball and socket approximation invalid. Functional calibration exercises do not take long, but they do add to the complexity of test protocols. It is possible that they may still have a role in people for whom palpation of pelvic landmarks is challenging, but these are also the people in whom soft tissue artefact is likely to be more problematic.

By contrast, functional calibration of the knee looks less promising. Lateral and medial epicondyles are generally reasonably easy to palpate, soft tissue artefact is known to be a specific problem with knee markers (Li et al. 2009; Tsai et al. 2009; Akbarshahi et al. 2010) and the hinge is assumed to be a poor approximation for even the healthy knee. Despite the apparent ease of palpation of the epicondyles, however, determining the true coronal plane of the knee is known to be a major challenge for gait analysis. This may, in part, be because few implementations of the CGM actually support the placement of calibration markers directly on the epicondyles. Both KAD placement and thigh marker alignment are technically more challenging than is often assumed. It may also be attributable to gait analysts being taught to concentrate on visualising the functional flexion–extension of the knee joint to guide thigh wand of KAD placement which is not at all easy.

The main aim of functional calibration of the knee is therefore to determine the alignment of the flexion axis on the assumption that this may give a more accurate representation of the transepicondylar axis and hence the coronal plane of the femur than the currently used techniques. Given that the screw home effect introduces transverse plane movement of the knee in the last 20° of extension to neutral and that knee markers are particularly prone to soft tissue movement with flexion of between 20° and 80° is probably optimal. Avoiding full extension in standing can be achieved by asking the patient to only extend until the toe comes in contact with the floor. A range of algorithms are available (Baker et al. 1999; Schwartz and Rozumalski 2005; Chang and Pollard 2007b; Ehrig et al. 2007). Anecdotal evidence has been encouraging, but little formal evidence has been presented to demonstrate benefits. The main problem is probably in identifying a criterion standard for validation purposes.

Early positive results from using functional calibration to distinguish talo-crural and subtalar joint axes of the ankle (van der Bogert et al. 1994) have not been replicated. Many people undergoing gait analysis have restricted movement at the ankle joint that would prevent use of such techniques even if they were successful in the wider population.

Best practice in the clinical application of functional calibration is probably that implemented at Gillette Speciality Children's Healthcare where both a conventional CGM and a variant incorporating function hip and knee joint calibration are implemented and the results compared. Agreement increases the confidence in the biomechanical modelling, whereas disagreement reduces it.

Upper body models

The sophisticated models of the upper extremity that are currently being developed are rarely needed for clinical gait analysis. The arms have much less mass than the trunk and legs and are generally subjected to quite modest accelerations. Whilst they do contribute to the overall dynamics of walking, this effect is quite small and unlikely to be significant in the context of clinical interpretation. It can be useful to have an overall impression of upper extremity posture, but this can be achieved with relatively simple marker sets and will not be discussed further.

The trunk is different. The term *passenger unit* (Perry 1992) accurately identifies trunk movement as almost entirely a consequence of the way the limbs move and the moments exerted upon it by the hip muscles. It does not, however, convey how the heavy mass of the trunk has a major effect on the dynamics of walking. This is particularly important in many pathological gait patterns in which the trunk is moved in such a way as to compensate for a range of impairments. Allowing the trunk to lean laterally, for example, can move its mass more directly over the hip joint centre and reduce the hip abductor moment as a compensation for weak hip abductors. Some children with spina bifida use this mechanism extremely efficiently to allow walking even though they have minimal hip abductor strength. To understand such mechanisms, it is essential to have some understanding of how the trunk is aligned. (Having said this, most clinical gait analysis is based on pattern recognition rather than detailed understanding of the underlying biomechanics in which case measurement of trunk movement may not be so critical.)

A number of models have been proposed (Leardini et al. 2009), but a consensus has not emerged as to which is preferred. A major issue is how to handle deformation within the trunk. Some models consider the trunk as a single segment, whereas others model the thorax separately to the pelvis. Modelling the whole trunk may give a better impression of its overall alignment and therefore give a better reflection on the probable dynamic effects, but modelling the thorax separately is obviously required if any appreciation of movement within the trunk is important. Several early models (Davis et al. 1991; Bartonek et al. 2002) located markers on the shoulder girdle, which may move with respect to the thorax if there is marked upper extremity movement during walking as in some conditions. More recent studies (Nguyen and Baker 2004; Leardini et al. 2011) have tended to place the markers on the mid-line of the thorax and these should be preferred (see Figure 4.4).

Although the C7 vertebra is most prominent, it moves markedly with the neck and T2 is the preferred location. The line from this to a marker at T10 then defines the primary (vertical) axis of the thorax. Rotation about this can be defined by a marker on the centre of the

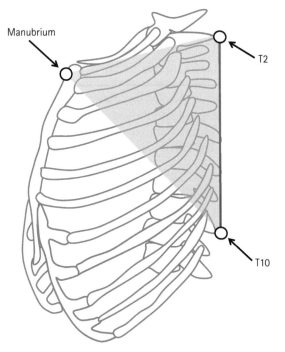

Manubrium

T2

T10

Figure 4.4 Minimum markers for an axial thorax model. The mid-point of the posterior superior iliac spine (PSIS) markers can be used instead of T10 for a segment representing the whole trunk rather than just the thorax.

manubrium. Placing a marker on the xiphoid process is also possible (Leardini et al. 2011). A T-shirt can normally be taped reasonably easily to allow the T2, T10 and manubrium markers to be visible. It can be slightly trickier to do this discretely for the xiphoid process marker in adolescent girls or women. If a measure of overall trunk alignment is required, then an equivalent segment can be defined using the T2 and manubrium along with the mid-point of the PSIS markers.

Foot models

As far as gait biomechanics is concerned, the foot is the interface between the body and its environment. In many conditions, including cerebral palsy, a poorly functioning foot is associated with reduced walking ability and often with an abnormal gait pattern. In order to understand the interaction between the foot and the rest of the body during walking, both measurements and a conceptual framework within which to understand them are required. A useful foot model will be one that provides that conceptual framework. The CGM models the foot as a single line rather than a full segment and cannot provide this. It is so widely applied though that many gait analysts do not even consider foot function beyond dorsiflexion of the ankle and foot progression.

Advanced modelling techniques such as forward dynamic simulation and induced acceleration analysis (see Chapter 5) are known to be highly sensitive to the small differences in how the foot is modelled. Whilst this can be seen as a criticism of those techniques, it also suggests that subtle impairment of foot function might be expected to have significant effects on gait. In complex multi-level conditions such as cerebral palsy, it is quite possible that these effects might be as significant as the more obvious proximal impairments.

Until fairly recently, few measurement systems were capable of detecting the positions of markers widely spaced over the whole body and multiple closely spaced markers on the foot. Modern systems can make such measurements, however, and the use of multi-segment foot models incorporated within lower extremity models is likely to become more common. A recent systematic review (Deschamps et al. 2011) found 15 multi-segment foot models reported in the literature. Although up to nine segments have been proposed, there is an emerging consensus in favour of just three or four segments. Few of the models have been used outside the centre they were first developed in and the discussion here will be limited to the Oxford Foot Model and IOR (Istituti Ortopedici Rizzoli) foot models which look likely to become the most widely available. The only other model that appears to have been adopted outside the centre in which it was developed is the Milwaukee foot model (Kidder et al. 1996; Johnson et al. 1999; Myers et al. 2004; Canseco et al. 2010; Long et al. 2010). This requires weight-bearing radiographs of the feet to calibrate the model to the bones within the feet. Whilst such an approach has clear advantages for patients with significant foot deformities, the practical challenges of arranging for radiographs to be taken on the same day as the gait analysis make it unlikely that this approach will be adopted for widespread clinical use. The Heidelberg Foot Measurement Method (Simon et al. 2006) has also been used in several centres. Whilst this defines anatomical angles that correspond to common radiological measurements, it is not based around specific segments and, as the name implies, should probably not be regarded as a 'model' (Baker and Robb 2006).

Oxford foot model

The Oxford Foot Model (Carson et al. 2001; Stebbins et al. 2006) comprises independent (6DoF) hindfoot and forefoot segments and uses a single marker to measure dorsiflexion of the hallux. (An independent tibia segment is also described, but this is superfluous if the tibia is being modelled as part of the rest of the lower extremity.) Markers on the posterior distal calcaneus (CAL1), over the sustentaculum tali (STAL) and opposite this on the lateral aspect of the foot (LCAL), are used to track the hindfoot segment (see Figure 4.5). An additional marker over the posterior proximal calcaneus (CAL2) is used for anatomical calibration in which the sagittal plane of the hindfoot is that containing markers CAL1, CAL2 and the mid-point of STAL and LCAL and the primary axis is the anterior axis which is defined as being in this plane and parallel to the floor in standing (if the person cannot stand with their foot flat on the floor then the primary axis is taken as being in the same plane but aligned with the projection of CAL1 and P5MT onto this plane).

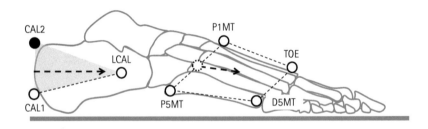

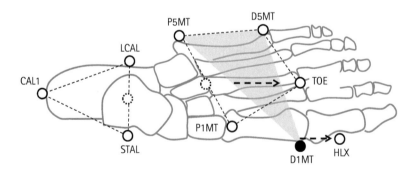

Figure 4.5 Lateral and superior views of the Oxford Foot Model. White-filled markers are used for tracking, black markers are used for calibration only. Grey triangles represent anatomical segments and the dashed lines indicate the principal axes. Dashed polygons link tracking markers for the different segments. (See text for descriptions of marker positions.)

The forefoot segment is tracked by markers placed laterally on the proximal and distal heads of the fifth metatarsal (P5MT, D5MT), superiorly on the proximal head of the 1st metatarsal (P1MT) and between the distal heads of the 2nd and 3rd metatarsals (TOE). The anatomical transverse plane is that containing P5MT, D5MT and a calibration marker placed medially over the distal head of the 1st metatarsal (D1MT). The principal axis is anterior defined as being the projection of the line from the mid-point of P5MT and P1MT to TOE (placed between the heads of the 2nd and 3rd metatarsals). The principal axis of the hallux is taken as being the line from D1MT to HLX The joint rotations describe the alignment of the principal axis of the distal segment with respect to the globe fixed in the proximal segment (see Chapter 2).

Istituti ortopedici rizzoli model
The IOR model is more recent (Leardini et al. 2007), but two repeatability studies (Caravaggi et al. 2011; Deschamps et al. 2012) have already been published and it is being implemented by a major software supplier. The foot is modelled as three independent three-dimensional segments plus six bi-dimensional segments (see Figure 4.6), with a subset of the tracking markers on each segment being used for the anatomical calibration. Several markers appear to be placed similarly to markers on the Oxford Foot Model, but there are often subtle distinctions, and therefore the different marker labels used in the original papers have been used (refer to the original publications for more detail).

The calcaneus segment is tracked by markers on the upper central ridge of the posterior surface of the calcaneus (CA), the lateral apex of the peroneal tubercle (PT) and the most medial aspect of the sustentaculum tali (ST). These also define the transverse plane of the segment. The primary (anterior) axis is defined as being from calcaneus to the mid-point of peroneal tubercle and sustentaculum tali. The metatarsus (forefoot) is tracked by markers on the base and heads of the 1st (FMB, FMH), 2nd (SMB, SMH) and 5th (VMB, VMH) metatarsals. The transverse plane of the overall anatomical segment

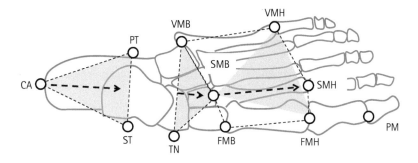

Figure 4.6 Superior view of the IOR Foot Model. Grey triangles represent anatomical segments and the dashed lines indicate the principal axis (lying in the planes defined by the triangles). Dashed polygons link tracking markers for the different segments. (See text for descriptions of marker positions.)

is defined by SMB, VMH and FMH and the anterior axis is the line from SMB to SMH projected onto this plane. The mid-foot segment is defined by a marker on the most medial apex of the navicular tuberosity and markers VMB and SMB. These three markers define the anatomical transverse plane, with the anterior axis directed from the mid-point of tuberosity and VMB to SMB.

Joint rotations are calculated differently to the Oxford Foot Model and the convention described in Chapter 2 in that the upward axis (rather than the anterior axis) of the distal segment is that which is described relative to the globe fixed in the proximal segment. The original article (Leardini et al. 2007) plots joint angles for five combinations of segments (which includes some redundancy), another seven angles describing the sagittal and transverse plane orientations of the hallux and individual metatarsals and a further angle describing the medial longitudinal arch.

References

Akbarshahi M, Schache AG, Fernandez JW, Baker R, Banks S, Pandy MG. Non-invasive assessment of soft-tissue artifact and its effect on knee joint kinematics during functional activity. *J Biomech*, 2010, 43:1292–1301. DOI: 10.1016/j.jbiomech.2010.01.002

Areblad M. *On modelling of the human rearfoot*. PhD, Linkoping Institute of Technology, 1990.

Baker R, Finney L, Orr J. A new approach to determine the hip rotations profile from clinical gait analysis data. *Hum Mov Sci*, 1999, 18:655–667. DOI: 10.1016/S0167-9457(99)00027-5

Baker R, Robb J. Foot models for clinical gait analysis. *Gait Posture*, 2006, 23:99–400.

Bartonek A, Saraste H, Eriksson M, Knutson L, Cresswell AG. Upper body movement during walking in children with lumbo-sacral myelomeningocele. *Gait Posture*, 2002, 15:120–129. DOI: 10.1016/S0966-6362(01)00147-3

Benedetti MG, Catani F, Benedetti MG et al. Data management in gait analysis for clinical applications. *Clin Biomech (Bristol, Avon)*, 1998, 13:204–215.

Camomilla V, Cereatti A, Vannozzi G, Cappozzo A. An optimized protocol for hip joint centre determination using the functional method. *J Biomech*, 2006, 39:1096–1106.

Canseco K, Rankine L, Long J, Smedberg T, Marks RM, Harris GF. Motion of the multisegmental foot in hallux valgus. *Foot Ankle Int*, 2010, 31:146–152. DOI: 10.3113/FAI.2010.0146

Cappello A, Cappozzo A, La Palombara PF et al. Multiple anatomical landmark calibration for optimal bone pose estimation. *Hum Mov Sci*, 1997, 16:259–274.

Cappello A, Stagni R, Fantozzi S, Leardini A. Soft tissue artifact compensation in knee kinematics by double anatomical landmark calibration: performance of a novel method during selected motor tasks. *IEEE Trans Biomed Eng*, 2005, 52:992–998.

Cappozzo A, Cappello A, Croce UD, Pensalfini F. Surface-marker cluster design criteria for 3-D bone movement reconstruction. *IEEE Trans Biomed Eng*, 1997, 44:1165–1174.

Cappozzo A, Catani F, Croce UD, Leardini A. Position and orientation in space of bones during movement: anatomical frame definition and determination. *Clin Biomech (Bristol, Avon)*, 1995, 10:171–178. DOI: 10.1016/0268-0033(95)91394-T

Cappozzo A, Della Croce U, Leardini A, Chiari L. Human movement analysis using stereophotogrammetry. Part 1: theoretical background. *Gait Posture*, 2005, 21:186–196.

Caravaggi P, Benedetti MG, Berti L, Leardini A. Repeatability of a multi-segment foot protocol in adult subjects. *Gait Posture*, 2011, 33:133–135. DOI: 10.1016/j.gaitpost.2010.08.013

Carson MC, Harrington ME, Thompson N, O'Connor JJ, Theologis TN. Kinematic analysis of a multi-segment foot model for research and clinical applications: a repeatability analysis. *J Biomech*, 2001, 34:1299–1307.

Chang LY, Pollard NS. Constrained least-squares optimization for robust estimation of center of rotation. *J Biomech*, 2007a, 40:1392–1400. DOI: 10.1016/j.jbiomech.2006.05.010

Chang LY, Pollard NS. Robust estimation of dominant axis of rotation. *J Biomech*, 2007b, 40:2707–2715.

Charlton IW, Tate P, Smyth P, Roren L. Repeatability of an optimised lower body model. *Gait Posture*, 2004, 20:213–221. DOI: 10.1016/j.gaitpost.2003.09.004

Collins TD, Ghoussayni SN, Ewins DJ, Kent JA. A six degrees-of-freedom marker set for gait analysis: repeatability and comparison with a modified Helen Hayes set. *Gait Posture*, 2009, 30:173–180. DOI: 10.1016/j.gaitpost.2009.04.004

Davis R, Ounpuu S, Tyburski D, Gage JR. A gait analysis data collection and reduction technique. *Hum Mov Sci*, 1991, 10:575–587. DOI: 10.1016/0167-9457(91)90046-Z

Della Croce U, Leardini A, Chiari L, Cappozzo A. Human movement analysis using stereophotogrammetry. Part 4: Assessment of anatomical landmark misplacement and its effects on joint kinematics. *Gait Posture*, 2005, 21:226–237. DOI: 10.1016/j.gaitpost.2004.05.003

Deschamps K, Staes F, Roosen P et al. Body of evidence supporting the clinical use of 3D multisegment foot models: a systematic review. *Gait Posture*, 2011, 33:338–349. DOI: 10.1016/j.gaitpost.2010.12.018

Deschamps K, Staes F, Bruyninckx H et al. Repeatability in the assessment of multi-segment foot kinematics. *Gait Posture*, 2012, 35:255–260. DOI: 10.1016/j.gaitpost.2011.09.016

Ehrig RM, Taylor WR, Duda GN, Heller MO. A survey of formal methods for determining the centre of rotation of ball joints. *J Biomech*, 2006, 39:2798–2809. DOI: 10.1016/j.jbiomech.2005.10.002

Ehrig RM, Taylor WR, Duda GN, Heller MO. A survey of formal methods for determining functional joint axes. *J Biomech*, 2007, 40:2150–2157. DOI: 10.1016/j.jbiomech.2006.10.026

Harrington ME, Zavatsky AB, Lawson SE, Yuan Z, Theologis TN. Prediction of the hip joint centre in adults, children, and patients with cerebral palsy based on magnetic resonance imaging. *J Biomech*, 2007, 40:595–602. DOI: 10.1016/j.jbiomech.2006.02.003

Hicks JL, Richards JG. Clinical applicability of using spherical fitting to find hip joint centers. *Gait Posture*, 2005, 22:138–145. DOI: 10.1016/j.gaitpost.2004.08.004

Johnson JE, Lamdan R, Granberry WF, Harris GF, Carrera GF. Hindfoot coronal alignment: a modified radiographic method. *Foot Ankle Int*, 1999, 20:818–825.

Kidder S, Abuzzahab F, Harris GF, Johnson JE. A system for the analysis of foot and ankle kinematics during gait. *IEEE Trans Rehabil Eng*, 1996, 4:33–38.

Kuo AD. A least-squares estimation approach to improving the precision of inverse dynamics computations. *J Biomech Eng*, 1998, 120:148–159.

Lamoreux L. *Errors in thigh axial rotation measurements using skin mounted markers*. Paper presented at the International Society of Biomechanics, 1991.

Leardini A, Benedetti MG, Berti L, Bettinelli D, Nativo R, Giannini S. Rear-foot, mid-foot and fore-foot motion during the stance phase of gait. *Gait Posture*, 2007, 25:453–462.

Leardini A, Biagi F, Belvedere C, Benedetti MG. Quantitative comparison of current models for trunk motion in human movement analysis. *Clin Biomech (Bristol, Avon)*, 2009, 24:542–550. DOI: 10.1016/j.clinbiomech.2009.05.005

Leardini A, Biagi F, Merlo A, Belvedere C, Benedetti MG. Multi-segment trunk kinematics during locomotion and elementary exercises. *Clin Biomech (Bristol, Avon)*, 2011, 26:562–571. DOI: 10.1016/j.clinbiomech.2011.01.015

Leardini A, Cappozzo A, Catani F. Validation of a functional method for the estimation of hip joint centre location. *J Biomech*, 1999, 32:99–103.

Leardini A, Sawacha Z, Paolini G, Ingrosso S, Nativo R, Benedetti MG. A new anatomically based protocol for gait analysis in children. *Gait Posture*, 2007, 26:560–571. DOI: 10.1016/j.gaitpost.2006.12.018

Li G, Kozanek M, Hosseini A, Liu F, Van de Velde SK, Rubash HE. New fluoroscopic imaging technique for investigation of 6DOF knee kinematics during treadmill gait. *J Orthop Surg Res*, 2009, 4:6. DOI: 10.1186/1749-799X-4-6

Long JT, Eastwood DC, Graf AR, Smith PA, Harris GF. Repeatability and sources of variability in multi-center assessment of segmental foot kinematics in normal adults. *Gait Posture*, 2010, 31:32–36. DOI: 10.1016/j.gaitpost.2009.08.240

Lu TW, O'Connor JJ. Bone position estimation from skin marker co-ordinates using global optimisation with joint constraints. *J Biomech*, 1999, 32:129–134.

Lucchetti L, Cappozzo A, Cappello A, Croce UD. Skin movement artefact assessment and compensation in the estimation of knee-joint kinematics. *J Biomech*, 1998, 31:977–984. DOI: 10.1016/S0021-9290(98)00083-9

Myers K, Wang M, Marks RM, Harris GF. Validation of a multi-segment foot and ankle kinematic model for pediatric gait. *IEEE Trans Neural Sys Rehabil Eng*, 2004, 12:122–130.

Nester C, Jones RK, Liu A et al. Foot kinematics during walking measured using bone and surface mounted markers. *J Biomech*, 2007, 40:3412–3423. DOI: 10.1016/j.jbiomech.2007.05.019

Nguyen TC, Baker R. Two methods of calculating thorax kinematics in children with myelomeningocele. *Clin Biomech (Bristol, Avon)*, 2004, 19:1060–1065. DOI: 10.1016/j.clinbiomech.2004.07.004

Perry J. *Gait analysis*. Thorofare, NJ, SLACK, 1992.

Peters A, Baker R, Morris ME, Sanqeux M. A comparison of hip joint centre localisation techniques with 3-DUS for clinical gait analysis in children with cerebral palsy. *Gait Posture*, 2012, 36:282–286. DOI: 10.1016/j.gaitpost.2012.03.011

Peters A, Sangeux M, Morris ME, Baker R. Determination of the optimal locations of surface-mounted markers on the tibial segment. *Gait Posture*, 2009, 29:42–48. DOI: 10.1016/j.gaitpost.2008.06.007

Piazza S, Okita N, Cavanagh PR. Accuracy of the functional method of hip joint center location: effects of limited motion and varied implementation. *J Biomech*, 2001, 34:967–973. DOI: 10.1016/S0021-9290(01)00052-5

Reinbolt JA, Schutte JF, Fregly BJ et al. Determination of patient-specific multi-joint kinematic models through two-level optimization. *J Biomech*, 2005, 38:621–626. DOI: 10.1016/j.jbiomech.2004.03.031

Sangeux M, Peters A, Baker RJ. Hip joint centre localization: evaluation on normal subjects in the context of gait analysis. *Gait Posture*, 2011, 34:324–328. DOI: 10.1016/j.gaitpost.2011.05.019

Schache AG, Baker R, Lamoreux LW. Influence of thigh cluster configuration on the estimation of hip axial rotation. *Gait Posture*, 2008, 27:60–69.

Schwartz MH, Rozumalski A. A new method for estimating joint parameters from motion data. *J Biomech*, 2005, 38:107–116.

Seay J, Selbie WS, Hamill J. In vivo lumbo-sacral forces and moments during constant speed running at different stride lengths. *J Sports Sci*, 2008, 26:1519–1529. DOI: 10.1080/02640410802298235

Simon J, Doederlein L, McIntosh AS, Metaxiotis D, Bock HG, Wolf SI. The Heidelberg foot measurement method: development, description and assessment. *Gait Posture*, 2006, 23:411–424. DOI: 10.1016/j.gaitpost.2005.07.003

Sommer H. A technique for kinematic modelling of human joints. *J Biomech*, 1980, 102:311–317.

Stebbins J, Harrington M, Thompson N, Zavatsky A, Theologis T. Repeatability of a model for measuring multi-segment foot kinematics in children. *Gait Posture*, 2006, 23:401–410. DOI: 10.1016/j.gaitpost.2005.03.002

Thelen DG, Anderson FC, Delp SL. Generating dynamic simulations of movement using computed muscle control. *J Biomech*, 2003, 36:321–328.

Thelen DG, Anderson FC. Using computed muscle control to generate forward dynamic simulations of human walking from experimental data. *J Biomech*, 2006, 39:1107–1115.

Tsai T-Y, Lu T-W, Kuo M-Y, Hsu H-C. Quanitfication of three-dimensional movement of skin markers realtive to the underlying bones during functional activities. *Biomedical Engineering: Applications, Bais and Communications*, 2009, 21:223–232. DOI: 10.4015/S1016237209001283

van der Bogert A, Smith G, Nigg BM. In vivo determination of the anatomical axes of the ankle joint complex: an optimisation approach. *J Biomech*, 1994, 27:1477–1488. DOI: 10.1016/0021-9290(94)90197-X

Yamaguchi GT, Zajac FE. A planar model of the knee joint to characterize the knee extensor mechanism. *J Biomech*, 1989, 22:1–10.

Chapter 5
Advanced processing techniques

Conventional clinical gait analysis has focused on joint angles, moments and powers as the primary outputs of the measurements made. There are, however, a rich variety of alternative methods for processing this data that have the potential to give considerable clinical insight, many of which have been explored in a research environment. For a number of reasons, muscle length and moment arm modelling appear to be the only such techniques that have been adopted into general clinical application, and this chapter focuses on these. Advanced kinetic techniques, such as forward dynamic simulations and induced acceleration analysis, appear to offer considerable potential to provide clinical insight; these are not yet used in routine clinical practice, however, and are not described here.

Advanced kinematic techniques

Muscle length modelling
Muscle length modelling is essentially a different way of presenting the kinematic data captured during gait analysis. Rather than outputting the data as joint angles they are used to estimate the length of individual muscles. The *muscle length* is defined as the distance between its origin on one bone and its insertion on another (Delp et al. 1990). The term has been criticised because what is actually reported is the length of the musculotendinous unit that comprises the length of the muscle and any tendon through which it acts. Some people in the field are justifiably concerned that this is an important distinction and that an alternative term should be used, but it is so widely accepted that this is unlikely to happen in the near future and the term will be used in this book.

The length of many muscles can be approximated, for the ranges of joint motion that occur during walking, as the straight line distance between the origin and insertion

Some other muscles, however, wrap around bones such as the psoas as it passes over the pelvis or are restrained by retinicular structures such as the flexor retinaculum of the foot. The simplest models incorporate such constraints using a *via-point* – a point through which the muscle is assumed to pass (Delp et al. 1990). In this case, the muscle length becomes the combined length of straight line sections from the origin through the via-points to the insertion (see Figure 5.1). It is also possible to develop more complex models in which the constraining surface is modelled in some way, and the length of a curved path around this is calculated (Charlton and Johnson 2001).

Whichever approach is used, the technique is dependent on assumptions as to where the origins, insertions and via-points are in relation to the underlying segments. These are specified as coordinates of these points relative to the segment coordinate systems. Software for Interactive Musculoskeletal Modelling (SIMM) was the first commercially available package to offer muscle length modelling (Delp et al. 1990; Delp and Loan 1995), and the coordinates used for the standard lower limb model supplied with it have become the most widely used for such modelling. These data are derived from 30 year old measurements on five cadavers mixed from two separate studies (Wickiewicz et al. 1983; Friederich and Brand 1990). Recent work (Arnold et al. 2010) based on

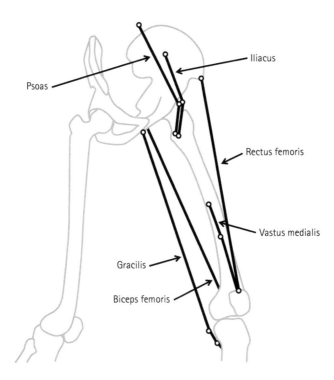

Figure 5.1 Modelling muscle lengths as straight line segments passing through specific via-points.

examination of 21 cadavers has led to a more definitve model which has been made publically available (www.simtk.org). It is important to note that muscle lengths calculated from these two models differ to an extent that may be clinically significant and thus results derived from the default SIMM model should not be compared directly with those derived from the new SIMTK model.

A variety of methods have been used to scale these data to people of different sizes. The earliest approaches simply used the joint angle output by another biomechanical model to drive this standard size model. More recent approaches have been similar but scale the muscle length model to the individual's height. A slight variant on this is to perform isometric scaling of each of the body segments independently according to estimates of their length from the static calibration measurements. For ease of clinical interpretation, these measurements then need normalising in some way, and perhaps the most common is to present them as a percentage of the length when standing in the anatomical position (with all joint angles set to zero).

One particular issue with muscle length modelling is that it is not appropriate to calculate lengths directly from either the conventional gait model (CGM) or the six degrees of freedom (6DoF) models. A subtle consequence of the way in which the CGM is defined is that the segments (particularly the femur and tibia) can vary in length as a consequence of soft tissue artefact, particularly of the lateral knee marker. If joint origins and insertions are scaled to this segment length, then their position will be subject to the same soft tissue artefact and it is impossible to determine how much of the change in muscle length is 'true' and how much is a consequence of this artefact. Although 6DoF models generally assume rigid body segments, similar soft tissue artefacts can lead to measured joint dislocations that are largely artefact and also corrupt the muscle length measures. In both modelling approaches, the joint angles are probably still reasonably reliable, and the most appropriate approach is to use these to drive a separate multi-link rigid body model to calculate muscle lengths. One advantage of the implementation of kinematic fitting techniques is that the same model that is used for kinematic fitting will also be appropriate for muscle length modelling.

Muscle length modelling is only really useful for a restricted range of muscles. The muscle length graph for a uniarticular muscle is extremely similar in shape to the relevant joint angle, and little information is gained by plotting both. Plotting the joint angle is generally more useful clinically because this is measured in degrees and can be compared directly with clinical examination measurements. This is illustrated in Figure 5.2 where the shape of the traces for the vasti lengths is extremely similar to the knee flexion angle both for the data plotted and for the reference data. There are minimal differences between the lengths of the two vasti and there is little point plotting both of these out. The data for the biarticular rectus femoris, however, are quite different from either the knee or hip flexion graphs. It would be extremely difficult to appreciate whether the rectus was long or short from the joint angle graphs alone.

It is also necessary to consider the characteristics of the model. Whilst the psoas is anatomically a multi-articular muscle, for example, most gait models only allow

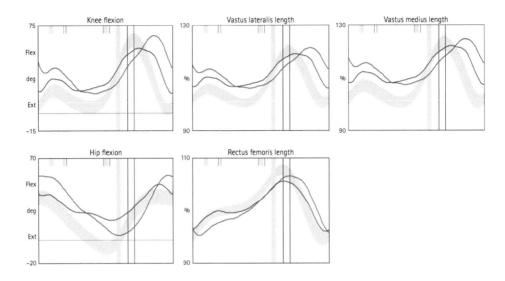

Figure 5.2 Illustration of muscle length modelling of uniarticular and biarticular quadriceps muscles (see text for commentary).

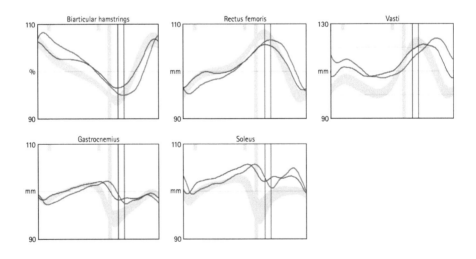

Figure 5.3 Typical output of the most useful muscle length data.

movement at one of those joints (the hip), and for modelling purposes it is best regarded as a uniarticular muscle. The muscles for which length modelling is particularly useful in clinical gait analysis are therefore the biarticular hamstrings, rectus femoris and gastrocnemius. Plotting the vasti and soleus alongside these for comparative purposes can also be useful (see Figure 5.3).

Some care is needed in interpreting muscle length data. Because of the source of the coordinate data, the limitations of isometric scaling and the presence of bone and joint deformity in many people, the measurements are more of an approximation than the joint angles from which they are derived. The other common mistake is to assume that because a muscle is short it must be tight. All that a short muscle indicates is that there is a reduced distance between the origin and insertion, which may be because a muscle is tight but may occur for a number of other reasons. The biarticular hamstrings during normal walking, for example, are shortest in early swing (see Figure 5.3) even though they are relaxed at this time and knee flexion is a passive phenomenon.

Muscle velocities

Spasticity has been defined as a 'velocity-dependent' phenomenon (Lance 1980), and therefore its effects might be expected to be observed in the rate of change of muscle length throughout the gait cycle (Arnold et al. 2006a, 2006b). This is known as muscle velocity. To get a true appreciation of muscle velocity, it is necessary to calculate the change in muscle length per unit time and plot the resulting variable on a gait graph (see Figure 5.4). The slope of the muscle length graphs gives an impression of muscle velocity, but this can be misleading because of the way that time normalisation scales all data to the duration of the gait cycle whether the walking is fast or slow. It should be noted that some authors have reported muscle velocity as the change in muscle length for a given percentage of the gait cycle, which suffers from the same limitations and should be avoided. In making conclusions about the effects of spasticity, this approach has the same limitation as muscle length in that it does not distinguish between length changes in the muscle and tendon.

Moment arm modelling

The same modelling approach can be used to calculate the moment arms of each muscle. In two dimensions, the moment arm of a muscle is the perpendicular distance

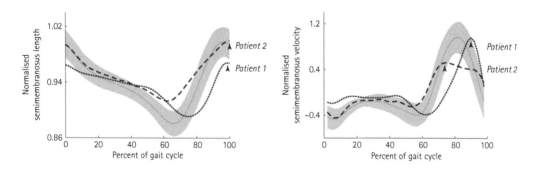

Figure 5.4 Muscle length and velocity graphs for the hamstrings of two patients with cerebral palsy. Data are normalised to the average normal maximal length or lengthening velocity (Figure from Arnold et al. 2006a with permission).

of a muscle's line of action to the joint centre. The moment that the muscle exerts is the multiple of this and the muscle force. It is possible to extend this concept to three dimensions to derive three quantities that represent the moment about the three axes of rotations divided by the magnitude of the applied force (Pandy 1999), but these moment arms are essentially abstract quantities and do not have an equivalent geometrical representation. They can be plotted on gait graphs and give an indication of any given muscle capacity to exert a moment about a joint. Unfortunately, they are even more sensitive to modelling and measurement error than the muscles lengths and are rarely used clinically.

References

Arnold AS, Liu MQ, Schwartz MH, Ounpuu S, Delp SL The role of estimating muscle-tendon lengths and velocities of the hamstrings in the evaluation and treatment of crouch gait. *Gait Posture*, 2006, 23:273–281. DOI: 10.1016/j.gaitpost.2005.03.003

Arnold AS, Liu MQ, Schwartz MH, Ounpuu S, Dias LS, Delp SL Do the hamstrings operate at increased muscle-tendon lengths and velocities after surgical lengthening? *J Biomech*, 2006b, 39:1498–1506. DOI: 10.1016/j.jbiomech.2005.03.026

Arnold EM, Ward SR, Lieber RL, Delp SL A model of the lower limb for analysis of human movement. *Ann Biomed Eng,*, 2010, 38:269–279. DOI: 10.1007/s10439-009-9852-5

Brand RA, Crowninshield RD, Wittstock CE, Pedersen DR, Clark CR, van Krieken FM. A model of lower extremity muscular anatomy. *J Biomech Eng*, 1982, 104:304–310.

Charlton IW, Johnson GR Application of spherical and cylindrical wrapping algorithms in a musculoskeletal model of the upper limb. *J Biomech*, 2001, 34:1209–1216.

Delp SL, Loan JP. A graphics-based software system to develop and analyze models of musculoskeletal structures. *Comput Biol Med*, 1995, 25:21–34.

Delp SL, Loan JP, Hoy MG, Zajac FE, Topp EL, Rosen JM. An interactive graphics-based model of the lower extremity to study orthopaedic surgical procedures. *IEEE Trans Biomed Eng*, 1990, 37:757–767.

Friederich JA, Brand RA Muscle fiber architecture in the human lower limb. *J Biomech*, 1990, 23:91–95.

Lance J. Pathophysiology of spasticity and clinical experience with baclofen. In: Feldman R, Young R, Koella W (Eds.), *Spasticity: Disordered motor control*. Year Book Medical Publishers, Chicago, 1980, pp. 485–495.

Pandy M. Moment arm of a muscle force. *Exercise and Sports Science Reviews*, 1999, 27:79–118.

Wickiewicz TL, Roy RR, Powell PL, Edgerton VR Muscle architecture of the human lower limb. *Clin Orthop* 1983, 179:275–283.

Chapter 6
Electromyography

In consultation with Adam Shortland

For a substantial period between the1960s and the mid-1980s, the only practical clinical gait analysis that was available was electromyography (EMG). Pioneers such as Perry and Sutherland in America and Baumann in Europe focused specifically on collecting and interpreting EMG signals. The reasons for this were practical; recording a small number of electrical signals on a chart recorder was the only technology available. All three clinicians experienced difficulty in interpreting EMG in the absence of kinematics and experimented with different ways of including movement data in their analyses. Perry developed observational techniques while Sutherland and Baumann used cine recording. Since the advent of commercially available motion capture systems, the focus in clinical gait analysis has shifted somewhat and most services now regard kinematic data as the primary data type and kinetics and EMG as secondary to this. In many laboratories, EMG is no longer regarded as one of the core measurements used for all patients and is only recorded when specifically requested or considered useful by the analyst.

Capturing good-quality EMG data is an art as well as a science and requires considerable attention to detail. Like many other techniques in gait analysis, it requires a good understanding of both the physiological function that is being measured and the scientific principles of the tools being used. Regular practice is necessary to develop and maintain the necessary skills. Appropriate training is also important. Capturing good-quality kinematics and kinetics is difficult enough, and it is unreasonable to expect someone who is learning this art to be learning to capture high-quality EMG data at the same time. It is therefore preferable to teach EMG at a different time.

The relegation of EMG to a secondary data source is a considerable problem. If EMG is only captured occasionally, then staff may not use the technique sufficiently to guarantee high-quality data collection when they do. Allocating patients that require EMG to a limited number of staff in order to ensure they develop and maintain this specialisation is one possible solution. Recording EMG as a standard procedure whether there is a clear clinical indication for it or not is another. Neither is particularly satisfactory. Regarding EMG as a secondary data source can also be problematic if it leads to a temptation to accept substandard EMG records. This can lead into a vicious circle if routine EMG data only get inspected superficially because staff are suspicious of its quality. This situation needs to be strongly resisted. If EMG data is to be captured, then it is essential that the highest standards of quality assurance are applied. If this is not the case, then it is probably not worth capturing the data in the first place.

The situation is probably exacerbated by some widespread practices in the way EMG data are collected, filtered and represented graphically. This chapter places a particular emphasis on describing techniques that augment efforts to ensure high data quality. One particular aspect here is to draw a distinction between the way data should be presented as part of the quality assurance process and, differently, as part of the clinical interpretation process.

The origin of the electromyography signal

Understanding how the EMG signal is produced in muscle can be extremely useful in understanding the principles on which good measurement technique is founded. Mammalian skeletal muscle is composed of fascicles that are bundles of muscle cells or fibres. In resting muscle, a negative electrical potential difference (–80mV) is maintained across the muscle cell membrane. When the nerve activates the fibre at the motor end plate, this reverses to a positive potential (+30mV) for about 2ms and this impulse, the *action potential*, travels along the length of the fibre at a speed of between 2 and 6m/s (see Figure 6.1). This generates a potential throughout the muscle and other tissues which gets smaller with distance from the depolarised section of the nerve. There will therefore be a difference in potential between the two electrodes as they are different distances away (d^+ and d^-). As the action potential comes under the first electrode (1) the signal detected gets bigger until just before it is under the first electrode (2) when the detected signal is at a maximum. When the action potential is between the electrodes, the difference between d^+ and d^- actually reduces until it is zero when at the mid-point (3) when the signal is zero. It continues to grow increasingly more negative until the action potential has just past the second electrode (4) after which it reduces in size as it moves away (5). The result is that the signal looks like a symmetrical pair of spikes. The timing between point 2 and point 4 will depend on the distance between the electrodes (D) and the conduction velocity. If the distance is 10mm and the conduction velocity is 4m/s then this will be 2.5ms. This is about the same time as the width of the spike in the action potential and hence of the spikes in the EMG signal.

Although this impulse has a total range of 110mV across the cell membrane, its effect falls off rapidly with distance in the immediate vicinity of the muscle, having reduced by 75% within the first 100μm from the cell membrane. The signal detected at the muscle

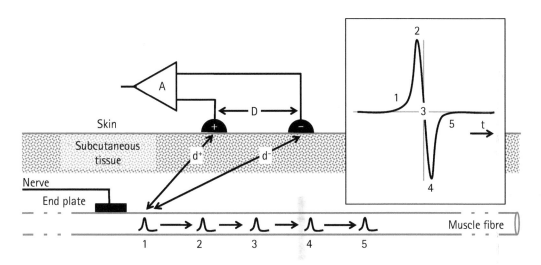

Figure 6.1 Schematic diagram of detection of signal from a single muscle fibre action potential. (See text for description.)

is determined by two factors. First, the signal reduces with distance. The thicker the skin and subcutaneous tissue the smaller the signal, and it is also clear that activity in more superficial fibres will be more readily detected than deeper ones. The greater impedance of thicker tissues also has a filtering effect, reducing the magnitude of the signal peaks. A typical peak-to-peak signal at the skin surface might be 5000µV (5mV) in a lean athlete but can be considerably less in others. The other factor that determines the signal magnitude is the distance between the electrodes. The larger this is, the larger the difference is between d^+ and d^- and hence the bigger the detected signal (for a given depth of muscle and other tissues). Unfortunately this is achieved at the cost of reduced specificity. The electrodes will pick up signals from a larger volume, and it is important that this does not include those from other muscles in the vicinity.

A number of different fibres are innervated by a single nerve and are therefore always activated together; this is described as a *motor unit*. Because the motor end plates are at differing locations on the different fibres, this can mean that a number of pulses can be travelling along parallel fibres with quite small time separations. This can lead to superposition of a number of signals such as depicted in Figure 6.1, and the combined effect can be a broadening of the spikes or the production of triphasic or even multi-phasic signals. These combine further with signals generated from fibres in other motor units so that the resulting signals are a dense sequence of spikes when the muscle is active, which diminish in both magnitude and frequency when the muscle relaxes (see Figure 6.2). Each action potential is of the same magnitude but those from fibres close to the skin will be attenuated less by soft tissues and appear larger in the EMG signal.

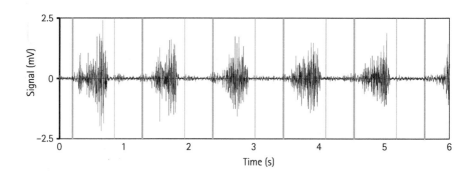

Figure 6.2 Good–quality raw EMG signal comprised of superimposed positive and negative spikes while the muscle is active and periods of much lower magnitude when the muscle is inactive. Grey vertical lines denote foot contact and foot off for five consecutive strides.

Equipment

Systems
There are now a number of high-quality EMG measurement systems on the market, and most of these are specifically designed to measure EMG during walking and similar activities. This reduces the requirement of the operator to understand the specific technical characteristics of the system, but these are outlined briefly below. The most practical change over recent years has been the development of wireless EMG units. These lead to considerable time savings through removing the requirement to tape down multiple cables. Specialist groups interested in investigating various aspects of latency have questioned whether the network protocols used by such systems have a sufficiently robust time-base, but this is not generally an issue for clinical gait analysis. The number of channels is also important. Around 12 or 16 channels allow a good range of muscles on both limbs to be measured. Anything less than this may reduce the choice of muscles that can be investigated or require separate measurements of, say, left and right sides.

Electrodes – surface
For clinical gait analysis, surface electrodes are generally adequate and to be preferred. Disposable gel electrodes are probably most commonly used and recommended by SENIAM[1] guidelines (Hermens et al. 1999). These have a silver electrode that makes contact with the skin through a silver chloride gel. The gel is surrounded by an annular foam pad coated with adhesive to attach it to the skin. The gel conductive area should be 10mm or less in diameter. Larger electrodes can give an increased magnitude of signal but decrease the frequency content and may be more susceptible to cross-talk from other muscles. Such electrodes are connected to the amplifier by snap connectors on short lengths of cable.

---

[1] SENIAM (Surface electromyography for the non-invasive assessment of muscles) was an influential European project to define guidelines for clinical EMG.

This wire is kept short as it has the potential to act as an aerial and pickup electromagnetic noise. Electrodes are applied in pairs typically about 2cm apart (centre to centre). Placing electrodes further apart may increase signal size but does so by detecting electrical signals from a wider volume and may introduce cross-talk from neighbouring muscles. For smaller muscles, the interelectrode distance may need to be even smaller. When positioning electrodes close together, care is needed to ensure that the gels do not connect.

The quality of gel electrodes is dependent on obtaining a low impedance across the electrode pair which can be checked with an Ohmmeter (values of 1–5KΩ are excellent and of over 30KΩ are concerning). Impedance can be reduced by shaving off any hair, lightly abrading the skin to remove dead skin and oils (fine abrasive paper tape for clinical use is now available – note that overuse of abrasive may lead to 'weeping' which may short out the electrodes) and cleaning with alcohol (which should be allowed to dry before placing the electrode). Well-prepared skin should take on a light pink colour.

An alternative is *dry* or *active* electrodes. In these, a pair of metal electrodes is built into a housing that also incorporates the electronics of the preamplifier. This construction allows amplifiers with a very high input impedance (~10TΩ) and low capacitance (3 or 4pF), which makes the sensor less sensitive to the quality (impedance) of the skin electrode interface. Skin preparation is less important and even shaving may not be required. The sensors are not self adhesive and therefore need to be taped to the skin. Artefact may arise if there is movement between skin and electrode, and firm circumferential taping may be required. A visible imprint of the electrodes should be anticipated upon removal of the tape. These will generally disappear within 10–20minutes but may occasionally last up to 24hours.

Electrodes – fine wire
Fine wire electrodes detect the signal between the tips of two very thin wires that are inserted into the muscle together and can be just a few millimetres apart. As a consequence, they pick up signals for only a small group of muscle fibres immediately around them. This can be an advantage for small muscles but in larger muscles the signal may not be representative of the muscle as a whole. For some deeper muscles, especially the tibialis posterior, surface EMG is simply not possible and fine wires are the only method for measuring EMG in these muscles.

There was a time when individual services would assemble their own fine wire electrodes. It is now virtually impossible to sterilise such assemblies to the levels required by current clinical best practice; so most services now buy these assembled and sterilised. Two fine wires (25–100μm diameter) made of a stiff highly non-oxidising metal (90% platinum – 10% iridium is commonly used) and insulated with Teflon or nylon are passed along the cannula of a hypodermic needle (see Figure 6.3). At the tip of the needle, short sections of the wires are bent back to form barbs. About 2mm of insulation is stripped from each wire and the electrical signal is detected between these two ends. It is important that these ends do not make contact with each other within the muscle, and making the barbs of slightly different lengths can help achieve this. At the other end of the wires, about 20mm of the wire is stripped of insulation to allow connection to the amplifiers.

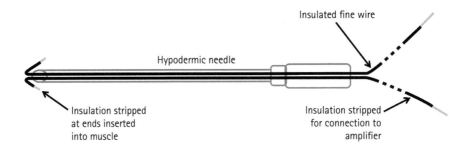

Figure 6.3 Fine wire electrode. (Dashed sections of wire indicate that there is a considerably greater length of wire than shown to allow connection to the amplifier.)

Once the insertion site has been selected and any local anaesthetic cream has had time to act, the needle is smoothly inserted and withdrawn to leave the electrode inserted in the muscle whilst measurements are made. The barbs will lodge at the deepest point to which the needle is inserted, so it is important not to go too deep during the insertion process. The wires are sufficiently flexible that they will straighten out on gentle pulling for removal. Care is therefore needed to ensure that no tension is applied to the wires after insertion either manually or as a result of muscle contraction. To check placement, a suitably approved electrical stimulation device can be attached to the electrodes. Starting at a low level, the stimulation can be slowly increased until a small twitch is noted in the required muscle. *Needle* electrodes are available in which a modified needle remains in place and serves as the electrode. These can be manufactured with extremely small interelectrode distances (which can go down to 25µm) and detect signals from very specific regions of muscle but are extremely sensitive to movement and are therefore rarely used in gait studies.

Signal processing

The electrodes are connected to amplifiers. The quality of the connection between electrodes and amplifiers is critical as any noise introduced into the system here will be amplified along with the EMG signal. High-quality connectors should be used, and it is generally preferable to leave sufficient slack on the connecting cables so that movement during walking does not apply stress to the connectors. Opinions differ as to whether taping down increases or decreases susceptibility to such movement artefact. The amplifiers also need to be of high quality. The input impedance of modern amplifiers can be greater than $10^{15}\Omega$ with a common mode rejection ratio of greater than 85 decibels. Most of the useful frequency content of the surface EMG signal is in the range 20–500Hz, and the amplifier obviously needs to cover this range (signals from fine wire electrodes contain frequencies up to 2000Hz). Gains of between 500 and 1000 are generally required. Notch filters to reduce the effects of AC mains frequency noise can remove useful signal information but are generally not required if high-quality amplifiers are used along with best practice in electrode placement. The signal is digitised using a sampling rate of at least twice the highest frequency content of interest so typically between 1000 and 2000Hz.

There are a variety of different opinions on how data should be presented for clinical interpretation. Many clinicians, aware of the potential for signal processing to conceal artefact, prefer to perform interpretation from the data as digitised (i.e. without further signal processing). Marking gait events (foot contact and foot off) on the EMG signals is clearly a minimum requirement for interpreting EMG in the context of gait analysis. This still means, however, that the format of the data is quite different from all the other data used in gait analysis which is time-normalised and plotted on gait graphs. Inspecting this 'raw' data is essential for quality assurance purposes but further signal processing results in data that more strongly augment the other graphical data.

The first stage of almost all signal processing is to apply a low-pass filter to remove any residual low-frequency movement artefacts in the data. In Figure 6.4, the raw signal has some evidence of minor artefacts when the muscle is inactive. The high-pass filter (at 20Hz) has removed these. This is followed by *rectification* of the signal. Whether the spikes from individual action potentials appear as positive or negative values is essentially random; so the average signal over any period should be close to zero. Converting all the minus values to positive values results in EMG 'activity' over any period having a positive value (see Figure 6.4). A filter can then be applied, which might be described as a moving average, integrating or envelope filter. Essentially all these calculate the average signal over a short period of time. This filters the individual spikes out to give a smoother 'envelope' reflecting the magnitude of EMG activity. The smoothness will depend on the frequency of the filter. A higher frequency filter will preserve more of the appearance of the original signal. A lower frequency filter will tend to smooth details out. The lower the frequency of the filter, the more it will reduce the magnitude of the peak signal. Using a zero phase delay filter is essential to preserve information about the timing of the signals.

A final stage used in some clinical services is to apply a threshold detection. In Figure 6.4, this has been applied to the 10Hz envelope filter. If the trace lies above the threshold value (the dashed horizontal line), then the muscle is recorded as on and if it lies beneath it then it is recorded as off. It can be seen that the apparent timing of muscle activity can be very sensitive to both the frequency characteristics of the filter and the level taken as the threshold relative to the signal magnitude. It is also apparent that a considerable amount of information is lost through applying threshold detection, and it is not at all clear why this method has persisted in clinical gait analysis for so long. Much more complex algorithms are also available to perform a similar task (Staude et al. 2001).

The signals can then be displayed on gait graphs in the same manner as any other gait variables (see Figure 6.5). It can be seen that the higher frequency filter gives more 'ragged' traces and more apparent variability from cycle to cycle. The lower frequency filter gives more apparent consistency from cycle to cycle. The lower frequency filter smoothes out the signal, resulting in a lower magnitude and differences in timing. The 20Hz filtered data, for example, appear to have ended just before toe off whereas the

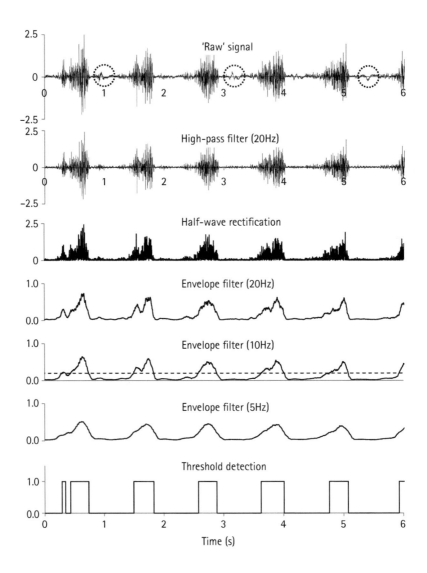

Figure 6.4 Different stages of EMG signal filtering. Dotted circles show small artefacts in the data. Note the scaling of the graphs changes as the envelope filters reduce the magnitude of peak signals. Threshold detection is performed on the 10Hz envelope filtered data, with the threshold represented by the dotted line on that graph.

5Hz filter smoothes the data out, suggesting there is still a small amount of activity after toe off. These differences are generally subtle, however, and the added clarity of the more consistent smoother graphs is probably to be preferred. Whatever decisions are made, it is obviously important that these are consistent between patients and also for any normative reference data that is used.

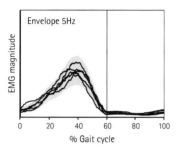
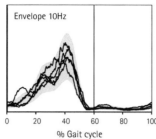
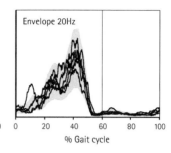

Figure 6.5 Gait graphs derived from electromyography data using three different envelope filters. The data are that illustrated in Figure 6.4 but could equally well represent cycles taken from different walks.

Normalisation

The amplitude of the measured signal varies with a large range of factors, many of which are not related to the level of EMG activity at all (thickness of skin and subcutaneous tissues, quality of skin preparation and separation of electrodes). The absolute magnitude of the signal is an important indicator of signal quality, and data for quality assurance purposes should be plotted on an absolute scale. For clinical purposes, however, the absolute magnitude is of much less significance, and plotting a signal normalised in some way can be useful. The most common method for this is to capture activity during a maximum voluntary contraction (MVC) for each muscle as part of the test protocol. Exactly how this is done will vary with the muscles being tested, but the general principle is that the person is given some sort of task during which they will activate the muscle as much as possible. The most common form is pushing or pulling against an immoveable object. The magnitude of signals captured during gait can then be presented as %MVC. This is not always appropriate as some people attending for gait analysis have difficulty eliciting and sustaining an MVC. One helpful feature, if this approach is adopted, however, is that there is no particular reason why the contraction has to be isolated. It is quite acceptable, for example, to measure the MVC in a child with cerebral palsy who is invoking a mass extensor pattern. Another approach is to normalise data to the highest signal measured during the test period. There is obviously little significance at all in the magnitude of signals normalised in this way, but this does optimise presentation of data to examine relative changes in magnitude. A variant of this is to ask the individual to walk as fast as possible and measure the maximum signal during this activity (den Otter et al. 2004; Schwartz et al. 2008). Data in Figure 6.5 have been normalised in this way.

Whether normalisation is appropriate and how it is performed will depend on the clinical condition of the person being analysed and the purpose of the analysis. Although normalisation to MVC is becoming more and more common in research, it has not been widely adopted in clinical practice. Many clinical packages automatically adapt scaling so that the data is scaled to fit the space available. This is essentially equivalent to normalisation to peak signal during activity, and this is probably the most common form of normalisation in clinical practice.

Quality assurance

Assuring the quality of EMG signals is relatively simple in principle. Most quality assurance tests require a consideration of the absolute magnitude of the signal. Software which auto scales the signal to fit the plotting area is extremely misleading and should be avoided during this activity. The first requirement is that the signal should be minimal when the person is relaxed and not activating any muscles. In healthy people with good-quality instrumentation and skin preparation, baseline signals of less than 2μV should be attainable. Obviously some people attend gait analysis for muscle disorders of various kinds, which preclude them from relaxing to this extent. Such people are relatively rare though, and it is worth spending a little time getting the person thoroughly relaxed for a short period after applying the electrodes in order to test the baseline signals. It can be extremely useful to record this signal for reference during clinical interpretation.

The next requirement is that the signal should increase significantly when the muscle is active. It is therefore important to ask the person to activate their muscles briefly against load shortly after applying each electrode. There is no particular reason for insisting on isolated activation of a particular muscle for this. Again a measure of absolute signal size is the best indicator of signal quality. It should be possible to get peak signals of several hundred microvolts from most muscles although smaller magnitudes are acceptable if the baseline signals are small. Even if an MVC is not to be used for normalisation, it is worth spending a little time capturing data during maximal activation.

A good-quality EMG signal looks like a dense sequence of spikes superimposed on each other when the muscle is active. (Figure 6.2 is a reasonably good example of this although the level of activity when the muscle is 'off' could be lower.) The spikes should also be distributed roughly symmetrically about the origin. As has been explained above, the width of these spikes is generally of less than 5ms duration, meaning that when plotted to fit a gait graph with an aspect ratio of 3:4 the individual spikes should have negligible width (the upstroke should be superimposed on the downstroke). Any feature that is broad enough for the rising and falling edges to be clearly distinguished is probably a consequence of artefact (examples can be seen in Figure 6.4). To check for such artefacts, it is essential to look at the raw signal as first digitised. (Figure 6.6 is an example of movement artefact that could easily be missed if the data have been high-pass filtered before checking.)

The next stage of quality assurance is to check for cross-talk. This occurs when activity in a muscle other than the target muscle is detected. It requires a series of carefully thought-out active tests to try and elicit muscle activity in one muscle group only in order to ensure that that activity is not being picked up by other electrodes. It can be difficult to achieve differential muscle activity in related muscle groups (e.g. the gastrocnemius and soleus), but it is possible for most muscles of interest in healthy

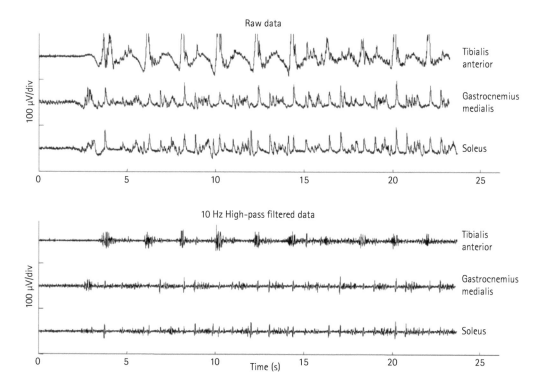

Figure 6.6 A borderline case of a meaningless signal, made out of rhythmic artefacts only, which could be misinterpreted as muscle activity after the application of a high-pass filter, set at 10Hz in this case (Figure from Merlo and Campnini 2010 with permission).

individuals. Again recordings of signals recorded during these tests can be extremely useful for reference if any doubts arise during the interpretation process.

Whether such tests are useful in patients with upper motor neurone disorders such as cerebral palsy or adult hemiplegia is questionable. In such people, co-activation of anatomically close muscle groups is exceedingly common. Evidence of differentiated muscle activity is indicative of selective electrode placement (and is useful), but it is impossible to distinguish whether cross-talk arises from poor electrode placement or genuine co-activation.

The final stage of quality assurance is to get the person to walk up and down a few times either observing live read-out on a computer screen or capturing some provisional data. Most people will show some degree of phasic muscle activity during walking, and this is the key feature that should be looked for in the data. Again looking at the absolute magnitude of signals can be extremely useful. The same indicators of the overall quality of the signal can be looked for as described above. It is during walking that movement artefacts are most likely to occur, and it is particularly important to look for these (again by reference to the raw signal). Movement artefacts are most often caused by loose or poor connections or electrode placements. They can also occur if connecting wires are too tight, exerting tension on connectors or other components. In people with known neuromuscular pathology, it is worth thinking through the expected patterns of EMG activity at this stage and comparing this with the observed signals.

Sensor placement and quality assurance exercises

Placing the sensors appropriately is the key to obtaining convincing EMG data The aim is to place the sensors on the muscle belly in line with the underlying fibres in such a manner that they are not also sensitive to cross-talk from adjacent muscles. Whilst rules for placement such as those suggested by SENIAM should serve as a guide for identifying the appropriate muscles, the precise placement needs to reflect the visible and palpable anatomy. This requires the analyst to understand why the particular locations are suggested. If the person is cooperative and able to do so, then asking them to selectively contract various muscles and move the joints allows a good impression to be gained of where the muscles are lying in that particular individual. In individuals with poor muscle development or excessive subcutaneous tissues, this may not be possible and more reliance on rule-based placements is inevitable.

It is important to remember that many conditions affecting those attending for gait analysis will lead to different muscle anatomy. It is well known that children with cerebral palsy, for example, often have shorter, less bulky muscles (Shortland et al. 2002; Fry et al. 2004; Barrett and Lichtwark 2010; Barber et al. 2011) often with longer tendons and which can be exaggerated after surgery (Shortland et al. 2004; Fryet al. 2007). These studies have tended to focus on changes to the internal architecture of muscle but clearly cannot exist without affecting optimum placements for electrodes. Ultrasound is becoming more commonly available within gait analysis services and can give valuable confirmation of appropriate sensor placement. More work is still required, however, to guide electrode placement in people with abnormal anatomy.

More advanced EMG techniques are now becoming available such as linear electrode arrays (Merletti et al. 2003), which have revealed areas of muscle termed *innervation zones* (Mesin et al. 2009). Electrodes placed symmetrically above such zones can pick up very small signals. These are best explained with reference to Figure 6.1. If the motor end-point was further to the right such as to be mid-way between electrodes d^+ and d^-, then an action potential will travel in both directions along the muscle fibre. The two potentials will have equal and effects on the opposing electrodes, and as such a potential difference will never exist between them and no signal will be measured. Whilst the existence of such zones is becoming more widely accepted, it is less clear as to how often bipolar electrode signals are affected in this way, exactly where they lie or how consistent they may be from individual to individual (Saitou et al. 2000). In principle, placing electrodes to avoid these zones is sensible, but this is little use if it is not clear where those zones are located. Given the current state of our knowledge, a pragmatic solution is required. If a particular electrode placement appears to give an abnormally low signal for no particularly good reason, then an innervation zone may be suspected, and moving both electrodes about 5–10mm in the same direction along the muscle fibres should be tried.

Quadriceps
The quadriceps are reasonably large and well-defined muscles. The rectus femoris passes in a more or less straight line from the ASIS to the superior pole of the patella and the vastus lateralis and medialis lie on either side. The sartorius passes obliquely from the ASIS to take a line medial to the vastus medialis and then down the medial thigh to insert on the proximal tibia The iliotibial band passes down the lateral thigh on top of the lateral portion of the vastus lateralis.

The distal rectus narrows and becomes tendinous towards the patella, and clearly electrode placement needs to avoid this section. Cross-talk with the medial and lateral vasti is minimised by a placement where the muscle belly broadens proximally. Cross-talk from the sartorius prevents too proximal a placement. SENIAM guidelines recommend a placement about 50% of the distance from ASIS to patella (see Figure 6.7). The electrodes should be aligned along the length of the muscle.

The vastus lateralis and medialis are both more bulky distally and combined with the slightly thinner rectus; this suggests a more distal placement. SENIAM guidelines for the vastus lateralis suggest placement about 66% of the distance from ASIS to

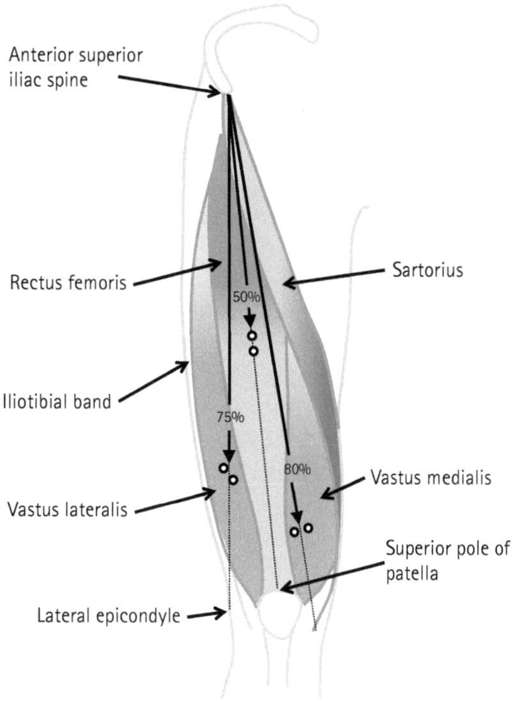

Figure 6.7 Sensor placement for quadriceps muscles.

the lateral side of the patella. The sensor could probably be even more distal and can also be placed more laterally. The only structure lateral to the muscle is the iliotibial band, which is entirely tendon at this level and is not a risk for cross-talk (although the signal magnitude may be reduced if the electrode is too lateral). It is suggested that 75% of the length of a tape measure wrapping round the surface of the thigh from ASIS to lateral epicondyle might be a more appropriate location. The fibres of the muscle run obliquely at this level, and the sensor should be orientated at about 45° to the long axis of the thigh.

Sensor placement for the vastus medialis needs to avoid the sartorius both medially and proximally. SENIAM guidelines suggest 80% of the distance from the ASIS to the 'joint space in front of the anterior border of the medial ligament'. A somewhat easier distal location to identify is the groove between the medial patella and the femur. At this point, the muscle fibres run almost transversely and the electrodes should be placed close to perpendicular to this line of reference.

Testing for the MVC of all the vasti is best achieved by knee extension against resistance (manual resistance of this will be difficult in healthy adults). With the placement suggested above, the main test required for cross-talk is to ensure that the rectus signal can be distinguished from either of the vasti. It is difficult to activate the vasti in isolation, but the rectus can be activated by resisting hip flexion whilst the knee remains relaxed.

Hamstrings
The lateral hamstrings and the long and short heads of the biceps femoris. The long head is generally a much bigger muscle lying over the short head and is likely to be the primary source of surface EMG signal. These muscles are bounded laterally by the iliotibial band. The two medial hamstrings (semitendinosus and semimembranosus) are smaller. The gracilis runs just medial of the semimembranosus for much of its length, with a section of the adductor magnus separating these proximally. The gluteus maximus runs across the hamstrings proximally covering the ischial tuberosity from which they all originate. All the hamstrings become tendinous distally.

The SENIAM guidelines are reasonably straightforward, with electrodes placed approximately half the distance from ischial tuberosity to the medial and lateral epicondyles, respectively, with the electrodes oriented along this line (see Figure 6.8). There is no attempt to separate out the two medial hamstrings muscles. In smaller children, it is questionable whether it is possible even to distinguish between the medial and lateral hamstrings group. MVC tests can be knee flexion against resistance in prone lying. Any cross-talk is likely to come between the muscles groups (which will be difficult to test for) or from the adductors medially; so carefully observing the signals during resisted hip adduction is a useful test.

Plantarflexors
The plantarflexors are also well-defined muscles. There is little evidence of differential activation between the medial and lateral head of the gastrocnemius, and EMG is often

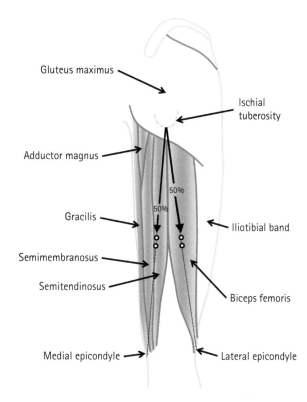

Figure 6.8 Sensor placement for the hamstrings muscles.

limited to the medial head (which is substantially bigger). A medial placement on the soleus avoids the possibility of cross-talk from the peroneal group.

Electrode placement is relatively straightforward (see Figure 6.9). SENIAM guidelines suggest placing the lateral gastrocnemius electrodes about a third of the distance from fibula head to the 'heel' and the soleus electrodes two-thirds of the distance from medial epicondyle to malleolus. Medial gastrocnemius placement is only described as on the 'most prominent bulge of the muscle'. MVC for all muscles is resisted plantarflexion. SENIAM guidelines suggest that this should focus on 'pulling the heel upward rather than the foot downward' but does not explain this further. It is difficult to preferentially activate gastrocnemius or soleus. Resisted knee flexion may activate gastrocnemius but not soleus. Performing mild active plantarflexion with the knee flexed might lead to preferential activation of the soleus.

Dorsiflexors and peroneal muscles
Tibialis anterior is a reasonably large muscle that is easily identified as lying just lateral to the crest of the tibia. The peroneals are much harder to distinguish from a group of muscles on the lateral aspect of the thigh including the tibialis anterior, extensor digitorum longus and the soleus. The peroneus brevis lies under the peroneus longus

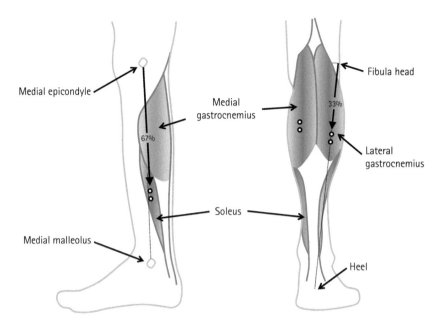

Figure 6.9 Sensor placement for the plantarflexors (medial and posterior views).

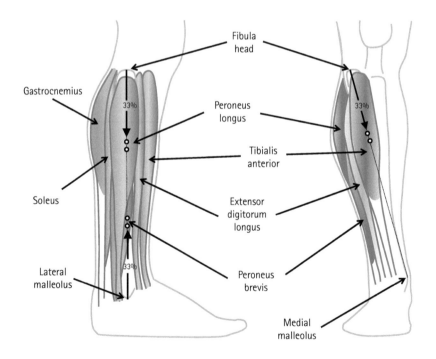

Figure 6.10 Sensor placement for tibialis anterior and peroneal muscles.

tendon and although SENIAM guidelines give recommendations for separate electrodes, considerable experience will be required to have confidence that activations will be detected separately from these two muscles (see Figure 6.10).

The placement for the tibialis anterior is a third of the way along a line from the fibula head to the medial malleolus. The exposed tibial crest gives some protection medially, and the electrode should be biased towards this side if anything. The peroneal electrodes are described as being one-third and two-thirds along the line from the fibula head to the lateral malleolus. The MVC of tibialis anterior is tested during dorsiflexion against resistance and that for the peroneals by eversion against resistance. Cross-talk should be looked for on the other channels when these exercises are being performed.

References

Barber L, Hastings-Ison T, Baker R, Barrett R, Lichtwark G. Medial gastrocnemius muscle volume and fascicle length in children aged 2 to 5 years with cerebral palsy. *Dev Med Child Neurol*, 2011, 53:543–548. DOI: 10.1111/j.1469-8749.2011.03913.x

Barrett RS, Lichtwark GA. Gross muscle morphology and structure in spastic cerebral palsy: a systematic review. *Dev Med Child Neurol*, 2010, 52:794–804. DOI: 10.1111/j.1469-8749.2010.03686.x

den Otter AR, Geurts AC, Mulder T, Duysens J. Speed related changes in muscle activity from normal to very slow walking speeds. *Gait Posture*, 2004, 19:270–278. DOI: 10.1016/S0966-6362(03)00071-7

Fry NR, Gough M, Shortland AP. Three-dimensional realisation of muscle morphology and architecture using ultrasound. *Gait Posture*, 2004, 20:177–182. DOI: 10.1016/j.gaitpost.2003.08.010

Fry NR, Gough M, McNee A, Shortland A. Changes in the volume and length of the medial gastrocnemius after surgical recession in children with spastic diplegic cerebral palsy. *J Pediatr Orthop*, 2007, 27:769–774. DOI: 10.1097/BPO.0b013e3181558943

Hermens HJ, Freriks B, Disselhorst-Klug C, Rau G. *SENIAM 8: European Recommendations for surface electromyography*. Roessingh Research and Development, 1999.

Merletti R, Farina D, Gazzoni M. The linear electrode array: a useful tool with many applications. *J Electromyogr Kinesiol*, 2003, 13:37–47. DOI: 10.1016/S1050-6411(02)00082-2

Merlo A, Campnini I. Technical aspects of surface EMG for clinicians. *The Open Rehabil J*, 2010, 3:98–109.

Mesin L, Merletti R, Rainoldi A. Surface EMG: the issue of electrode location. *J Electromyogr Kinesiol*, 2009, 19:719–726. DOI: 10.1016/j.jelekin.2008.07.006

Saitou K, Masuda T, Michikami D, Kojima R, Okada M. Innervation zones of the upper and lower limb muscles estimated by using multichannel surface EMG. *J Hum Ergol (Tokyo)*, 2000, 29:35–52.

Schwartz MH, Rozumalski A, Trost JP. The effect of walking speed on the gait of typically developing children. *J Biomech*, 2008, 41:1639–1650. DOI: 10.1016/j.jbiomech.2008.03.015

Shortland AP, Fry NR, Eve LC, Gough M. Changes to medial gastrocnemius architecture after surgical intervention in spastic diplegia. *Dev Med Child Neurol*, 2004, 46:667–673.

Shortland AP, Harris CA, Gough M, Robinson RO. Architecture of the medial gastrocnemius in children with spastic diplegia. *Dev Med Child Neurol*, 2002, 44:158–163.

Staude G, Flachenecker C, Daumer M, Wolf W. Onset detection in surface electromyographic signals: a systematic comparison of methods. *EURASIP J Adv Sig Process*, 2001, 2:67–81.

Chapter 7

Clinical video

In consultation with Adrienne Harvey and Jill Rodda

The availability of high-quality yet affordable camcorders for the consumer market opens up the possibility for almost anyone to make good-quality recordings of a person's walking. Almost all video footage taken in this way can be played back on a modern computer, and it is becoming increasingly straightforward to record directly to a computer. There are a number of relatively simple steps that can be taken to ensure good-quality video recordings for clinical use. Whether recording video on its own or in the context of a more complete instrumented gait analysis, it is worth investing some time in optimising conditions which can be summarised as

- Keep it bright
- Keep it big
- Keep it straight
- Keep it steady

Basic principles

Keep it bright
Perhaps the single most important factor in obtaining good video recordings is the quality of the light. If videos are to be recorded regularly in a given location, then installing good lighting is worthwhile. Having floodlights is one option but may be disconcerting for the patient and simply installing the best possible ceiling lighting is probably the best option. Florescent tubes give high light levels but can result in an irritating flicker when recording at high frame rates or with high shutter speeds. Tungsten bulbs give less light but also less flicker (simply installing more bulbs is a possibility). Modern halogen bulbs are probably the best option. Integral flash units on

some consumer camcorders are often ineffective particularly when the camera is some distance from the individual and are unlikely to improve image quality significantly. Any clinical gait analysis service recording video regularly, particularly if they are charging others for it, should obtain specific professional advice on how best to provide lighting.

A number of camera properties also affect the light illuminating the sensor. The most obvious is the lens size. The larger the aperture, the more light will be admitted to the sensor. Consumer camcorders tend to have fairly small apertures, and purchasing a camera at the low end of the professional range may well be a worthwhile investment for those regularly capturing clinical video. Camcorders also have a range of settings that affect illumination. Increasing frame rate and/or shutter speed will reduce the illumination. Standard frame rate of 25 or 30 frames per second is adequate for most clinical purposes (higher frame rates are only really required if running is being analysed), but shutter speeds of 1/125th or 1/250th second may be required to obtain good-quality stills from the video. Increasing the aperture and gain can compensate for low light levels but increasing the gain may give rise to more noise on the image. Most modern camcorders have good semi-automatic setting adjustment, and setting frame rate and shutter speed and letting the camera do the rest is often all that is required.

Keep it big

The aim should be to make optimum use of the field of view, and this can be controlled for by using the zoom on the camera. Wherever possible, optical zoom should be used as the digital zoom reduces the pixel resolution of the image. In normal walking, a person's stride length is about 80% of their height. The aspect ratio (ratio of height to width) of a conventional video image is 3:4. This represents a field of view 1.7 strides wide fitted to the height of the individual and hence for the full body to be captured for a full stride (see Figure 7.1). Widescreen format has a ratio of 9:16, which allows capture of the full body for a stride and a half. This makes it virtually certain that a full left or right stride will be captured for each walk, which can be extremely useful.

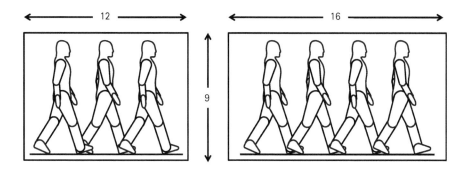

Figure 7.1 Format with 9:16 aspect ratios (right) allow more strides to be captured than 3:4 (9:12) aspect ratio (left).

Most clinical conditions result in reduced stride length; so generally more strides than this will be captured for patients. It is a good idea to start each session with a shot of the patient standing, and this allows the zoom to be adjusted to fit the height of the patient.

Keep it straight
An ideal clinical video would give a pure sagittal or coronal plane view of the patient. The camera should therefore be set up perpendicular to the relevant plane. Even then there is only a true sagittal or coronal plane view at the centre of the field of view. Anywhere else on the field of view, the patient will be recorded as if they are walking at a small angle to the camera – a phenomenon called parallax (Hillman et al. 1998; Brown et al. 2008). This gets worse the further the patient is from the centre of the field of view but improves the further the camera is from the patient (see Figure 7.2). Restricting the field of view to small number of strides therefore reduces parallax. Table 7.1 summarises the parallax at the edge of the field of view (1.5m from the centre) for different camera distances. It can be seen that moving the camera back to 8m or so reduces parallax considerably, but further improvements are more modest beyond this.

Unfortunately the amount of light received from the individual reduces with the square of the distance. There is therefore a need to compromise between the requirement to reduce parallax at the same time as keeping a bright image. The best solution is to ensure optimal lighting and then move the camera back whilst maintaining a good-quality image. Some testing may be required prior to collecting a clinical video to work out what this distance is. It is assumed here that as the camera is moved back, you zoom in to maintain the height of the individual. There is little point moving the camera further back beyond the capacity of the zoom to achieve this. In many practical situations, it will be the dimensions of the room that dictate how far back the camera can be positioned.

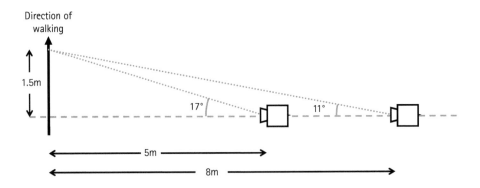

Figure 7.2 Diagram showing how parallax effects decrease as the camera is moved further away from the patient (1.5m represents one stride for a healthy adult).

Table 7.1 Effect of parallax 1.5m from the centre of the field of view, with the camera at different distances from the patient

Distance from camera (m)	Parallax at 1.5m from centre of field of view
3	27°
4	21°
5	17°
6	14°
8	11°
10	9°
12	7°

Keep it steady

Another key feature of good clinical video is keeping the camera steady, which requires the use of a tripod. Having a tripod that allows the camera height to be adjusted easily and with a head that allows for pan and tilt for fine tuning the orientation of the camera is useful. Some centres find that taking close-up footage of the feet is valuable, and the best images will be obtained if the camera is very close to the floor. If this is the case, then some care is needed in selecting a tripod as only a few allow this degree of adjustment.

Capturing video simultaneously with or separately from gait data

Recording clinical video is valuable in its own right (Harvey and Gorter 2011) but is also important in clinical interpretation of data from instrumented gait analysis. Details such as foot deformities are not captured well by current models, and video may be the best tool for observing these. Use of walking aids, orthoses and footwear is obvious from video which can prevent oversights or correct errors in recording the conditions under which instrumented gait data were captured. Facial expressions and overall body posture can suggest whether 'usual' walking is being observed or not. It is sometimes possible to see changes in muscle or tendon definition, which might suggest whether muscles are active or not. Video recordings can also be important for assuring quality of kinematic data, which should help explain what is observed on video but should not contradict it.

Many gait analysis systems allow the capture of synchronous video with other data from one or more cameras. Doing so has advantages and disadvantages. The most obvious advantage is that exactly the same walk is being captured, which is particularly important if there are discrepancies between video and other data. Sometimes being able to see marker placement on the video can either support or question whether they have been placed appropriately. Taking only simultaneous video will also save time and may protect the patient from undue fatigue.

There are disadvantages. Motion capture facilities generally require a central walkway, and few laboratories are big enough to allow video cameras to be far enough away from the individual to eliminate parallax effects under these conditions. Some motion capture systems perform less well under the high levels of illumination that are required for good-quality video, and some systems may not be capable of capturing data from higher resolution video cameras (although neither of these is a serious problem with the most recently available systems). Sometimes the location of markers may be misleading. Judging pelvic obliquity in the absence of markers can be difficult, for example, and if anterior superior iliac spine (ASIS) markers are visible but incorrectly placed, then the analyst may be drawn to erroneous conclusions by those markers (which of course will be supported by the kinematic data).

To obtain the best quality clinical video, it is probably best to record data separately to the gait data. If simultaneous video capture is available though, it is sensible to record this as well for quality assurance purposes.

Setting up the room for clinical video capture

Finding the space to record clinical video is often one of the most significant practical challenges. Ideally the space should be uncluttered, quiet and available for the sole purpose of the recording. Children are particularly prone to distraction if there is other activity in the room. Good-quality video requires space. It takes a couple of strides from standing for a person to establish a cyclic walking pattern and another couple to slow down and stop. The minimum requirement for good video over 2 strides is therefore 6 strides, which requires a walkway about 8m in length for a healthy adult (although many patients will require less). Considerably longer walkways will be required if jogging or running is to be recorded. To reduce parallax in sagittal plane recordings, a perpendicular distance of about 8m from walkway to camera is optimal. This is rarely possible, but 5m should be regarded as the minimal distance from the camera. The minimum room size for good video recording is therefore about 8m by 5m.

This requires the walkway to be along one wall and if a room is to be used regularly for this process, it can be useful to mark a walkway (about 0.8m wide) on the floor either with tape or by the use of different coloured floor covering. The background should be as uncluttered as possible where it can be seen by the camera. Recording against a plain wall is preferable. The extent of the wall that the camera sees can be quite small; so this need not be extensive (see Figure 7.3). Using floor and wall colourings that contrast with skin tones is preferable; green or blue are popular choices. Lighter colours may reflect too much light, which can make it difficult to obtain appropriate exposure for the patient. In a rectangular room set-up for capturing clinical video, there is considerable dead space that is not seen by the cameras that can be used for a variety of purposes.

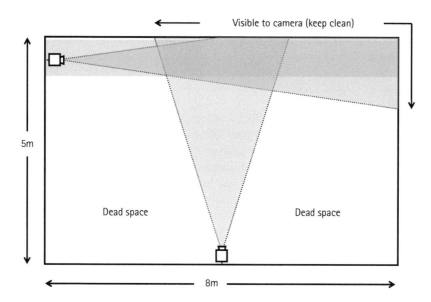

Figure 7.3 Minimum space for obtaining a good clinical video.

Placement of the camera for sagittal plane video is reasonably straightforward. Parallax will be minimised in the vertical direction if the camera is placed at about hip height (approximately half of total height) and the camera points horizontally forwards. Some more subtle factors affect coronal plane video. True parallax is much less of an issue because the patient remains central to the field of view. The key issue is left to right comparisons and with hips about 15cm from the mid-line, parallax is less than $3°$ even when the patient is as close as 3m from the camera. The bigger issue is that the patient will appear bigger as they move closer to the camera. Again the further the camera is from the indivdual, the smaller the change in size as the patient walks forwards through a given distance. The best strategy is probably to adjust the zoom such that the patient is viewed at full height when standing in the middle of the walkway. If the camera is at hip height pointing horizontally forwards this means that both the head and feet will be cropped as the patient walks in front of this point. As good footage of the feet is generally more useful than that of the head and shoulders, it can be a good idea to have the camera at a lower position than for the sagittal plane camera and angled slightly upwards to capture the full height of the patient in the middle of the walkway.

If there is only one camera, then there are clearly two options for recording coronal plane video after sagittal plane. The first is to have the patient move in the same direction but move the camera; the second is to maintain the camera position and ask the patient to walk in a perpendicular direction. Neither is inherently better, and the choice is largely personal preference though it might be influenced by the size and nature of the capture space and the type of patient being analysed (it might be easier for some patients to continue to repeat the same task rather than change to another one). Using two cameras either synchronously or at different times leads to the most efficient recordings.

'Special effects'

The easiest way to take good-quality clinical videos is to have static cameras mounted on appropriate tripods. It is possible to track the walking individual in the sagittal plane by panning the camera Motorised panning units are available, which can track the individual smoothly (but often take a little practice to operate proficiently). This means that more of the walk can be recorded, but recordings away from the centre of the walkway can be subject to considerable parallax and this needs to be kept in mind when interpreting recordings. A few centres have cameras mounted on a trolley or rails, which can be either pushed or are motorised. By keeping the camera parallel to the patient, the parallax can be kept to a minimum In both techniques, it can be difficult to perceive walking speed and how the patient is moving through space.

It is also possible to use the zoom lens so that the patient remains at a similar size during coronal plane recording. This can have the effect of losing focus as the patient moves, although some motorised zooms allow the focus to be tied to the zoom to prevent this. This can be a particular issue if close-up coronal plane views of the feet are recorded. Autofocus on camcorders can sometimes be affected by the movement of feet, particularly in close-up coronal view, and it may be necessary to disable this function for such shots and rely on manual focus instead.

If panning or zooming is used to keep the patient in a particular area of the field of view, then a video 'mixer' can be used to combine the video signals from two cameras such that the simultaneously recorded coronal image appears on the left half of the screen and the sagittal image on the right half of the screen This gives a very nice record for clinical purposes (although the need to keep the patient away from the centre of the field of view leads to moderately increased parallax effects). Unfortunately, there are no off-the-shelf packages available to deliver such functionality, and such systems are therefore beyond the resources of most centres. (Where such systems are available they are often designed for security camera installations, and it is important to note that the security cameras themselves rarely have the features required for capturing good-quality clinical video.) Simultaneous recording of separate signals from two cameras is becoming much easier either through a movement analysis system or through one of a number of stand-alone PC-based video capture packages. This gives flexibility to view recordings simultaneously or separately and is probably the most practical solution at present.

Equipment

Video cameras vary immensely in price. At one level, any camera is better than no camera, and if resources are scarce then a cheap consumer camcorder is a perfectly acceptable starting point (although it is important to check that any camera for clinical use can be mounted on a tripod). There are considerable advantages in purchasing a middle- or top-range consumer camcorder or even one at the lower end of the professional range. More expensive cameras tend to have larger aperture lenses and larger sensors. Both of these produce better quality images for a given light level. They will also tend to have better quality lenses to improve image quality. Frame rates higher than 25 or 30 frames per second do not add greatly to clinical video, but the ability to shutter at 1/125th or 1/250th second can be really useful to get good-quality stills when the video is paused. More expensive cameras will also offer higher resolution, but there is no real point in capturing video with higher resolution than the device on which the video will be viewed; digital video (DV) resolution is probably adequate for most clinical purposes.

If capturing to a storage device within the camera, then a remote control unit can be useful to allow one person to control the camera whilst remaining in close proximity to the patient. For routine clinical use, a mains power supply to which the camera connects directly can be extremely useful to avoid the risk of running low on battery power. Transferring images easily to a computer is important but is very simple in most modern camcorders either with a removable memory card or with a cable connecting directly to the computer (generally a USB or FireWire/IEEE 1394 connection). To capture directly to the computer, FireWire connectors on both cameras and computers are useful (a computer with two FireWire ports will be required to capture video simultaneously from two cameras).

Most modern personal computers come with the basic software to support capturing digital video and basic editing of clips. If you want to record from just one camera at any one time, then such packages are perfectly adequate. More complex packages are only required if you want to record simultaneously from multiple cameras.

Clinical protocols

It is a good idea to develop a fixed protocol for capturing clinical video. The gait analyst in charge of the capture session should always remain alert, however, for extra footage that may be of particular relevance for any individual patient's gait problems. Generally speaking, footage will be required in coronal and sagittal (from left and right) views for some combination of footwear, orthoses and walking aids (this will be described as a 'condition' throughout this book). Each specific condition increases the time required, however, which can be a particular issue if patients are prone to fatigue or loss of concentration. It is therefore sensible for each service to focus on two or three of conditions and for the analyst to clearly understand the rationale for selecting these. One condition might therefore be walking in bare feet with usual walking aids, which gives a good indication of the patient's underlying capacity. If he or she is able to manage short distances without aids, it might also be useful to capture this. Another condition would be the patient's most usual combination of footwear, orthoses and walking aids. Sometimes the focus of the analysis is to compare performance under different conditions, and clearly this will require a longer session. One limitation of video is that repeated viewing of the same recording can suggest more consistent walking patterns than are characteristic of the patient, and recording at least two walks from the principal camera angles can protect against this somewhat. If standard procedure specifies just one view, then the analyst should be particularly vigilant to ensure that this is representative of the general pattern of walking and repeat the capture if not (and record what has happened).

Typical protocol with motorised cameras
The standard protocol for clinical video at the Hugh Williamson Gait Laboratory (HWGL) in Melbourne was

1. Split screen view (full person sagittal on left, full coronal on right, Figure 7.4a),
2. Sagittal full body only (Figure 7.4b),
3. Sagittal waist down (Figure 7.4c),
4. Close-up of feet (Figure 7.4d, this is not part of the HWGL protocol but is used by several other services),
5. Coronal full body (Figure 7.4e),
6. Coronal mid-tibia down (Figure 7.4f).

For each of these, the patient walked up and down the full length of the walkway. Capturing the patient standing, initiating walking, turning and eventually stopping again were seen as important to augment the information gained from the majority of footage of natural walking. The sagittal camera panned with the patient and the coronal camera zoomed (with automatic adjustment of focus).

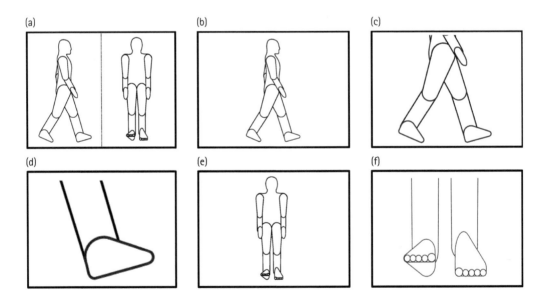

Figure 7.4 Storyboard representation of video sequence following the Hugh Williamson Gait Laboratory, Melbourne clinical protocol, with (a–c) panning of sagittal camera and (d–f) zoom of coronal camera.

Typical protocol with fixed cameras

It is not practical to capture close-up data in the sagittal plane with fixed cameras as it becomes more difficult to capture the part of the gait cycle required within the fixed field of view of the camera and in the coronal plane because of the difficulties of maintaining focus. Starting, stopping and turning at the ends of the walkway cannot be captured unless the patient is specifically requested to perform these actions in the field of view of the cameras.

A standard protocol with fixed cameras filming both coronal and sagittal planes simultaneously might be

1. Patient standing in the centre of field of view; zoom adjusted to height of patient (and focus if not using autofocus),
2. Patient walks forwards (gait initiation),
3. Turns and walks back full walkway,
4. Turns and walks back full walkway,
5. Turns, walks to middle of walkway, then turns and walks back,
6. Turns and walks back full walkway,
7. Turns, walks to middle of walkway, then turns and walks back,
8. Turns and walks back full walkway,
9. Turns and walks back to middle of walkway and stops.

This is depicted diagrammatically in Figure 7.5. It results in recording of two walks from each side, two turns, starting and stopping in a reasonably efficient manner.

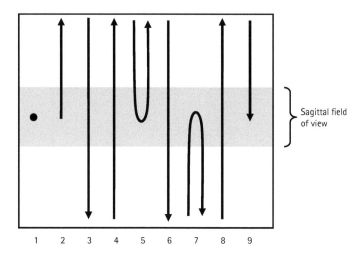

Sagittal field of view

Figure 7.5 Sequence of walking, turning and stopping to obtain good-quality clinical video with fixed cameras.

Protocol for videoed physical examination

It can be extremely useful to video parts of the physical examination. A shortened clinical examination can be videoed with the use of a chair as follows:

1. Patient stands facing the camera, with the femurs pointing forwards. Three coronal views are taken: full height (Figure 7.6a), from mid-thigh to feet (Figure 7.6b) and close-up of ankles and feet (Figure 7.6c). Patient turns to left and lifts the limb closest to the camera (with support if necessary) to provide close-up of medial aspect of weight-bearing foot (Figure 7.6d) and then turns through 180° and repeats for the other side.

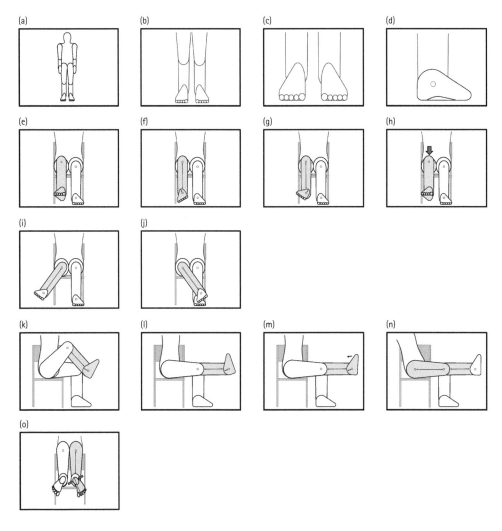

Figure 7.6 Storyboard representation of a simplified clinical examination for video recording. (See the text for full explanation.)

2. Patient sits on the chair facing the camera. Free active movement of the ankle into dorsiflexion (Figure 7.6e), eversion (Figure 7.6f) and inversion (Figure 7.6g) is recorded. Confusion test can be demonstrated (Figure 7.6h). Passive internal (Figure 7.6i) and external (Figure 7.6j) range of hip rotation is demonstrated in sitting.

3. Patient turns to sit sideways on the chair with sagittal view of right side. The knee is then flexed to 90° and passive range of dorsiflexion is demonstrated (Figure 7.6k), the knee is then extended to full range of extension whilst resisting dorsiflexion (Figure 7.6l). A fast Tardieu stretch (Figure 7.6m) can also be applied to demonstrate any signs of spasticity. Selective motor control of the ankle is shown by free active dorsiflexion with the knee extended. Passive knee extension is then recorded for knee fixed flexion deformity of the knee or hyperextension (Figure 7.6n). During this testing, it will sometimes be necessary for the patient to lean back a little and extend the hip if the hamstrings are tight. If safety in this position is a concern, a parent or staff member should stand behind the child.

4. The patient turns to sit the other way across the chair and the same tests applied to the left leg.

5. The patient is then asked to high kneel on the chair facing away from the camera which is zoomed in to give a close-up of the plantar surface of the foot, which might show callosities or foot deformity. Both malleoli are pointed to with the fingers to give an indication of tibial torsion (Figure 7.6o). Ideal alignment of the patient is with the femurs vertical and the tibias perpendicular to the camera.

References

Brown CR, Hillman SJ, Richardson AM, Herman JL, Robb JE. Reliability and validity of the Visual Gait Assessment Scale for children with hemiplegic cerebral palsy when used by experienced and inexperienced observers. *Gait Posture*, 2008, 27:648–652. DOI: 10.1016/j.gaitpost.2007.08.008

Harvey A, Gorter JW. Video gait analysis for ambulatory children with cerebral palsy: why, when, where and how! *Gait Posture*, 2011, 33:501–503. DOI: 10.1016/j.gaitpost.2010.11.025

Hillman SJ, Hazlewood ME, Loudon IR, Robb JE. Can transverse plane rotations be estimated from video tape gait analysis? *Gait Posture*, 1998, 8:87–90. DOI: 10.1016/S0966-6362(98)00028-9

Chapter 8

Physical examination

In consultation with Pam Thomason and Jill Rodda

A thorough standardised clinical examination is an integral part of any comprehensive clinical gait analysis. Although many health professionals are trained to conduct a semi-quantitative physical examination to guide their own clinical practice, gait analysis requires a quantitative examination that is sufficiently robust to inform someone else's clinical practice. Conducting an examination to this level of rigour is a highly specialised skill and will generally require considerable specialised training of new staff. In order to ensure the quality of the physical examination therefore, it is virtually essential that it is carried out by a staff trained and managed within the gait analysis service. Given this, it is almost universal for the clinical examination to be conducted at the same appointment as the gait analysis. The downside of this is that a physical examination conducted by such highly specialised staff is extremely expensive. This will be exacerbated if the examination takes place in the gait analysis space and prevents other use of the expensive measurement equipment and floor-space. If gait analysis services perform the physical examination as an integral part of any gait analysis, then purchasers are entitled to expect a high-quality product.

Given how central the physical examination is to a range of clinicians, the evidence base to support its implementation is generally quite poor. At a time when all other clinical measurement techniques and outcome scales are subjected to rigorous validation studies, there are very few studies of even simple measures of variability, such as the standard error of measurement (SEM), for even the most common physical examination measures. McGinley et al. (2009) in reviewing repeatability studies of gait analysis suggested that SEM of greater than 5° should be viewed as concerning but reached the conclusion that the evidence suggested that most clinically important joint kinematic measures can be made more precisely than this (McGinley et al. 2009). Studies reviewing SEM (McDowell et al. 2000; Fosang et al. 2003) for passive joint range of movement suggest that few fall within that range. It is also commonplace for gait data to be interpreted against explicitly defined normative data. It is quite difficult to obtain normative ranges of physical examination data from the literature, particularly for children, and few services are as particular about collecting normative physical examination data as they are for gait data.

It is important to remember that the physical examination is being conducted primarily for comparison with gait analysis data. Measurements should generally be made in a way that is consistent with the biomechanical model that is being used for gait analysis. This may require modification of some tests. The most obvious being that of the Thomas test for hip flexion contracture by positioning the pelvis such that the anterior superior iliac spine (ASIS) is vertically above the posterior superior iliac spine (PSIS). It is also important to note that if tests are modified, then results may not be directly comparable with those of the original tests. The Thomas test modified as described above will record about 10–15° more hip extension than the conventional test. If results are being released to external clinicians, it is important that this is made clear (in this case the test should be referred to as 'modified Thomas test').

Conducting a physical examination as part of a gait analysis is a compromise. There are an almost endless list of potentially useful clinical measurements, most of which can be measured at varying levels of sophistication and instrumentation. The examination, however, has to be fitted into a practical time-scale. When working with children, the primary limitation is their concentration span particularly if they have to co-operate with a full gait analysis afterwards. A balance also has to be struck between standardisation of the examination, which guards against omission of a core data, and customisation of the examination to ensure that tests that might be particularly important for a specific individual can be incorporated. In principle allowing considerable freedom for the gait analyst to customise the examination to the needs of the patient appears to be the best way to exploit the skills of a highly trained staff, but in practice this is a demanding task. Most services perform a standard set of core measurements in a systematic fashion but expect analysts to perform specific additional tests in addition to these if the patient's needs or condition requires this.

Adhering to a systematic protocol for core measurements has several advantages. It is one of the best ways to guarantee that all the core measurements have been recorded. Systematically working through an assessment is likely to reduce data entry errors. This can be particularly important if one person is making measurements and another is recording them. Working out a set protocol of tests grouped by the positioning requirements of the patient, which is well understood by the analyst and any assistant, is also important to obtain optimum use of the time available.

Physical examination data should be entered directly into electronic recording systems. These need not be complex but should allow for data to be entered in the order in which the tests are most efficiently performed and then output in a format that makes clinical and biomechanical sense. Figure 8.1 illustrates output grouped by the different muscle groups in a completely different order to that in which the tests are performed. Such recording systems can also incorporate some error checking to flag data with unexpected

	Left	Right
Hip extension (standardised Thomas)	0°	0°
Hip flexor strength	4+(2)	4+(2)
Hip extensor strength (knee 0°)	4+(2)	4(2)
Hip extensor strength (knee 90°)	4+(2)	4(2)
Hip abduction range (hip 0, knee 0)	23°abd	25°abd
Hip abduction range (hip 0, knee 90)	31°abd	34°abd
Hip abductor strength	4(1)	4(1)
Hip internal rotation range	87°int	83°int
Hip external rotation range	9°ext	5°ext

	Left	Right
Femoral anteversion	43°int	46°int

	Left	Right
Knee extension range (capsule)	0°	0°
Conventional popliteal angle	50°flex	46°flex
Standardised popliteal angle	54°flex	54°flex
Hamstrings spasticity (mod. Tardieu pop.)	56°flex	65°flex
Knee flexor strength	5(2)	5(2)
Knee extensor strength	4(2)	4+(2)
Quadriceps lag	0° flex	0° flex
Rectus length	112°flex	105°flex
Rectus spasticity (mod. Tardieu)	64°flex	73°flex

	Left	Right
Dorsiflexor strength	4(1)	4(1)
Confusion (+/−)	pos	pos
Dorsiflexion (knee 90°)	12°pf	4°df
Dorsiflexion (knee 0°)	15°pf	10°pf
Plantarflexor spasticity (mod. Tardieu)	23°pf	19°pf
Plantarflexor tone (mod. Ashworth)	3	3
Plantarflexor strength (knee 90°)	NT(NT)	NT(NT)
Invertor strength	4(1)	4(1)
Evertor strength	3(1)	5(1)

	Left	Right
Tibial torsion	13°ext	15°ext

	Left	Right
Thigh-hindfoot angle	12°ext	6°ext
Hindfoot-forefoot angle	3°ext	4°ext
Ankle equinus/calcaneus	normal	mild equinus
Hindfoot valgus/varus	normal	mild varus
Planus/cavus	normal	mild cavus
Forefoot abd/add	mild adductus	mild adductus

Weight (kg)	31	
Height (cm)	140	
True leg length (cm)	73	74
Apparent leg length (cm)	78	79

Figure 8.1 Formatted physical examination grouping measures related to hip, knee ankle and foot. Values in blue denote bone and joint deformities, in yellow denote muscle length, in orange denote muscle strength and in green denote neurological signs.

values such as abnormally high values, or values that appear inconsistent with other elements of the examination or with the diagnosis.

A rigorous physical examination is much easier to complete with an assistant. Many tests require a combination of stabilisation, patient handling and measurement, which can only be performed rigorously by two people. The analyst must be a properly accredited health service professional qualified to take responsibility for the examination. The assistant can be a technician from a broad range of backgrounds but needs to be trained to perform specific roles for the different tests. Practices vary between services as to exactly how roles are allocated, but examination remains the responsibility of the health professional. If the assistant is allocated the task of data entry, then they should be fully trained in this. Data entry errors are particularly likely if the person entering the data has little understanding of their meaning or importance.

Physical examination measures can be broadly divided into four categories: bone and joint deformity, muscle length, muscle strength and neurological signs. The remainder of this chapter is divided into sections describing the different types of tests and then a detailed description of commonly used tests described in an order that minimises the need to reposition the patient. A consideration of how physical examination measures relate to the gait data is discussed in Chapter 10.

Goniometer measurement

Many of the measures are of angles, and it is worth reviewing some of the principles of goniometry. An angle can be defined in terms of three points (one proximal, one distal and a common point). In this case, the goniometer axis needs to be placed over the common point and the arms directed towards the proximal and distal points. An angle can also be defined as the connection between two lines (one proximal and one distal). By definition, there is only one place that the goniometer axis can be placed in order that the two arms lie along the different lines. In this case specifying where the axis is placed is unnecessary and will almost always introduce ambiguity in how the measurement is to be made and should be avoided. Dorsiflexion, for example, is the angle between the lateral border of the plantar surface of the foot and the long axis of the tibia The analyst should aim to place the two arms of the goniometer along these lines, and when this has been achieved the goniometer axis will, by definition, be in the correct place. It is almost always easier to adopt this technique than to place the axis in a specific location (over the lateral malleolus in this case) and place the distal arm so that it appears to be parallel to the specified line.

In physiotherapy textbooks, it is common to see a focus on the 'starting' position for any test and then a description of the movement that is required. It is important to stress that it is the end-point that is primarily important for measurement. This is conceptually important for tests where the alignment of one segment is standardised. In the modified Thomas test, for example, it is important that the ASIS are directly above the PSIS after the stretch has been applied rather than before. This book will refer to 'position' rather than the 'starting position'. It is important to make sure that the overall body alignment is specified and that the patient is observed to be in this position when the measurement is taken This will be most important for the segments immediately adjacent to the joint being measured but measurements for multi-articular muscles can be influenced by the alignment of other segments as well.

As stated above, it is important that goniometer measurements are consistent with the biomechanical model used to generate joint kinematics. There is a balance here, however, as the models are generally defined in terms of joint centres that cannot be palpated. Making measurements truly consistent with the model may well introduce more subjectivity than basing them on easily identifiable bony landmarks. A pragmatic approach is required with tests defined in terms of bony landmarks unless this is likely to introduce large discrepancies with the biomechanical model.

It is useful to have a range of goniometers available and to use them appropriately. Good-quality plastic goniometers with scales subdivided to at least 2° increments are recommended. The larger the goniometer the easier it will be to read and the less guesswork will be required in positioning the arms along the long bones. Smaller goniometers, particularly those with straight edges, can be particularly useful for measuring dorsiflexion and for some other measurements on smaller children. Semicircular goniometers with one arm that can lie on the assessment couch can be particularly useful for providing a reference from which to measure the hip's internal and external rotation.

There is considerable variability across gait analysis services in the precision to which clinical examination data are recorded. Reliability studies tend to suggest that the SEM (McDowell et al. 2000; Fosang et al. 2003) of passive joint range is of the order of 5°, and it is sometimes assumed that there is no point measuring joint range to a higher precision. Rounding error, however, is an additional source of error. Imagine a child who really has 3° dorsiflexion range. If the SEM is 5° then, by definition, measurement of 8° or higher will be recorded on 17% of occasions. If this is rounded to the nearest 5°, then it could be recorded as 10°. Although it does not make statistical sense to *interpret* differences of less than the SEM, it is sensible to *record* measurements to greater precision. Most manual goniometers have 1° or 2° divisions, and it makes sense to record measurements to this precision. As a further example, consider a child who has pre- and postintervention measurements of 2° and 3°. If these are recorded to the nearest degree, then there is clearly no clinically significant difference. If these are rounded to 0° and 5°, then there will be a temptation to interpret this as a mild evidence of change.

It is common for a test to be performed quickly and informally to check whether the results are *within the normal limits* before performing a formal test with a measurement, with the result being indicated by some appropriate abbreviation (e.g. *wnl*). This can save time and allow for a focus on more relevant tests, but unless time is particularly constrained it should be considered a departure from best practice. Physical examination measurements recorded as part of gait analysis are often collated for audit or research purposes, and use of such a practice can invalidate even very basic statistics such as the mean and standard deviation. If a test is not performed for any reason, it is important that this is clearly indicated on the form (it is particularly important that software does not allocate a default value such as zero). It is also intriguing that although recording a measure as within normal limits is a widespread practice, there is very small amount of data regarding what such normal limits are.

Bone and joint deformity

Measures of bone and joint deformity are generally fixed geometrical properties of the skeletal system which do not vary with positioning or muscle activity. It is still important, however, to ensure that the patient is positioned in the correct position to allow the measurement to be made as specified. Joint deformities are included with bony deformities because they can be difficult to distinguish without reference to medical imaging. Several standard measures need minor modifications to make them compatible with kinematic measures. One particular issue is that common gait analysis models assume that the primary axis of the long bones links the proximal and distal joints and makes no account for deformation within the bone. Coronal plane bowing within the tibia, for example, is not taken into account.

Measures of torsional deformations of the long bones are also important particularly for the analysis of children with cerebral palsy. Anteversion is considered as the angle between the femoral neck axis and the knee joint axis when both are projected onto the transverse plane of the femur. Tibial torsion is similarly defined as the angle between the knee and ankle joint axes when both are projected onto the transverse plane of the tibia. Measures of the alignment of different parts of the foot are also important both in weight-bearing or on the couch.

Muscle length

In this book, *muscle length* is used to refer to the combined length of the muscle and any associated tendons (muscle belly and tendon length will be used to refer to the different components if necessary). Most measures of passive joint range of motion are, essentially, estimates of the length of the relaxed muscle and hence an indication of muscle contracture (Keenan et al. 2004). Biarticular muscles are somewhat more complex, with muscle length depending on the positions of two joints. Generally one joint is held in a standardised position and the range of movement of the other is measured. Some modifications to conventional clinical tests are required to make them more compatible with gait data such as performing the Thomas test with the pelvis position standardised. These tests can give different results to the conventional measures, and the use of modified tests should always be explicit when reporting results.

Methods for assessing passive joint range of movement are generally well understood by physiotherapists and other clinicians. The aim is to apply a stretch to the muscle whilst eliciting as little muscle activation as possible (definitive testing of muscle length is only possible when conducted under general anaesthesia). A considerable moment should be applied during the stretch for two reasons. The first is that moments exerted during walking are considerable, and the physical examination aims to inform interpretation of the gait data. The second is that the gradient of passive musculotendinous unit length with applied load increases at high load, and therefore measures of passive muscle length become less sensitive to the magnitude of the applied load.

Muscle strength

Following the National Institutes of Health Taskforce on Childhood Motor Disorders, *muscle strength* is defined as the ability *to generate normal voluntary force in a muscle or normal voluntary torque (moment) about a joint* (Sanger et al. 2006). In practice, it is the ability to generate a moment that is assessed. True moment-generating capacity is dependent on the muscle length and contraction velocity as well as on the inherent properties of both muscle and tendon. Instrumented measures for isokinetic (constant contraction velocity) or isometric (constant muscle length) are possible using various dynamometers, but these are generally too time consuming for use in combination with gait analysis. Hand-held dynamometers have been used for isometric strength testing in combination with research gait analysis. Several repeat measurements and careful positioning for different tests have been assumed to be important for making reliable measurements, and the additional time for these has generally excluded such techniques in combination with clinical gait analysis.

Most services, however, restrict strength measurement to manual muscle testing. This is variously attributed to Kendall (Kendall and Kendall 1949) or described as the MRC (Medical Research Council 1943) or Oxford Scale. It grades muscle strength on a 6-point scale (see Table 8.1), with Grade 3 representing the ability to overcome the effect of gravity on distal segments and Grade 5 representing normal strength. Despite being widely accepted, it has considerable problems biomechanically. The grading is supposed to be through the muscle range, whereas since Huxley's earliest experiments on muscle we have known that muscle strength varies considerably through its range. This is exaggerated in many children with cerebral palsy as illustrated by the quadriceps lag test which is essentially dependent on the ability to overcome gravity being dependent on joint angle. It is exacerbated by the fact that the effect of gravity of the distal segments in generating a moment about the joint changes as they move through the range of motion.

The other major limitation of the 6-point scale is that the major lower limb muscles in walking do not generally act against the effect of gravity on the distal segments, they act against the effects of gravity and inertia on the proximal segments (Fosang and Baker 2006; Dallmeijer et al. 2011). A Grade 3 hip flexor exerts a moment roughly equal to that required during normal walking, but a Grade 3 plantarflexor exerts less than 1% of that required (Fosang and Baker 2006). A further problem with assessing the plantarflexors is that in stronger individuals the maximum strength exerted may be

Table 8.1 Grades of muscle strength

Grade	Description
0	No muscle contraction detected
1	Flicker of activity but not sufficient to cause movement even when gravity is eliminated
2	Muscle can be moved when gravity is eliminated
3	Muscle can be moved against gravity
4–	Muscle can be moved against gravity and slight resistance
4	Muscle can be moved against gravity and moderate resistance
4+	Muscle can be moved against gravity and strong resistance
5	Full muscle strength. In adults, the examiner will have great difficulty resisting movement. Some subjective judgement will be required in distinguishing between 4+ and 5

O'Brien (2010).

limited by the analyst's ability to provide resistance. Various supplementary methods have been suggested to assess plantarflexor strength (Lunsford and Perry 1995) but none is particularly satisfactory.

Subdivision of gradings is common but applied inconsistently. Some authors suggest subdivisions should reflect the range of movement of which strength is available (Clarkson 2000; Paternostro-Sluga et al. 2008) rather than intermediate strength levels that are especially confusing. Recent versions of the MRC guidelines (O'Brien 2010) recommend subdivision of level 4 only as described in Table 8.1.

A further consideration is the degree to which muscles can be activated independently. Biomechanically, there is some justification in seeing this as quite separate to strength (see the section below on neurological signs), but it can equally be argued that having moment-generating capacity is largely irrelevant if you have no control over when the muscle is activated. A compromise is first to grade maximum muscle strength regardless of how this is achieved but then include selectivity in parenthesis afterwards, with 2 representing isolated activation, 0 representing activation only as part of a pattern involving other muscles and 1 as an intermediate grade.

Some assessors are concerned that patients can generate moments about one joint as a consequence of 'trick' activations of muscles at other joints, and this may lead to misleading muscle strength measures. This is virtually impossible during essentially static muscle strength testing (although patients do sometimes exploit multi-body dynamics to achieve movement at one joint by exerting a moment at another during walking and other activities). The only 'tricks' that needed to be guarded against are related to alignment. Clearly if alignment changes, then activation of one muscle group might look like an activation of another. A person cannot use their hip flexors to abduct the hip, for example, but by rotating the pelvis back they can make hip flexion look like hip abduction.

Neurological signs

There are several aspects of the physical examination that are assessed by testing muscles but are actually indicators of how the nervous system is functioning. These phenomena are complex and poorly understood (throughout medicine and biology), and there is little consensus on the definitions of even some of the most basic terms (Malhotra et al. 2009). The role of gait analysis is essentially that of identifying the impairments that are limiting walking and the focus of a physical examination for gait analysis is therefore on *spasticity*, *tone* and *selective motor control* as they affect specific muscle groups. The gait analyst should also be aware of broader categories of movement disorders such as *dystonia, ataxia, apraxia, dyspraxia, athetosis* and *rigidity*. Formal diagnosis of these requires a specialist neurological assessment for which patients should be referred if required.

The framework proposed by the National Institutes of Health Taskforce on Childhood Motor Disorders (Sanger et al. 2003, 2006) is probably most useful for distinguishing between the different neurological signs relevant to gait analysis. Following the earlier definition by Lance (1980), *spasticity* is defined as *resistance to externally imposed movement with increasing speed of stretch and varies with the direction of joint movement* (Sanger et al. 2003).[1] *Tone* is defined *operationally as passive stretch while the patient is attempting to maintain a relaxed state of muscle activity* (Sanger et al. 2003). The distinction between spasticity and tone is therefore whether the stretch is applied quickly (spasticity) or slowly (tone). *Selective motor control* is defined as *the ability of the body to isolate the activation of muscles in a selected pattern in response to demands of a voluntary posture of movement* (Sanger et al. 2006).

The Modified Ashworth Scale (Bohannon and Smith 1987) was initially described as a measure of spasticity but whether it is or not is dependent on the speed at which the test is performed. In the original paper, it was suggested that the movement should be performed through the full range of movement over a period of *about one second*. This is reasonably fast, too fast to be a test of tone, but falls short of lengthening velocities occurring during walking which generally occur within specific phases of the gait cycle (typically less than ¼ second). It is therefore not fast enough to be a useful test of spasticity that might be triggered during the gait cycle. In many gait analysis services, the assessment is performed at a slower speed as a measure of tone rather than spasticity. Tone is then graded on a 6-point scale as outlined in Table 8.2. As with other tests that are modified for gait analysis purposes, this should be made clear to clinicians who may be interpreting the results.

The Modified Tardieu Test (Boyd and Graham 1999) is a measure of spasticity which, being recorded as an angle, is convenient for gait analysis. In this test, which is a much simplified version of Tardieu's original proposal (Tardieu et al. 1954), muscle length is assessed first using the procedures outlined above, performing the stretch slowly. The test is then repeated performing the movement *as fast as possible*. If spasticity is present then the joint will catch at a specific angle and it is this that is reported as the result of the test. It is common to repeat the stretch three times to get a feel for the catch and make a measurement on the final stretch. In the absence of spasticity, the Modified Tardieu angle will be the same as the muscle length angle. The larger the difference between the two angles the greater the spasticity is assumed to be. This is, however, an oversimplification. If spasticity is really a velocity-dependent phenomenon, then the catch would be predicted to occur at a particular velocity rather than at a particular angle. Of course the joint is being accelerated in the test (its velocity is increasing with increasing angle), and the angle of catch might be an indirect measure of stretching velocity. We might therefore expect the results of the test to be sensitive to how vigorously the test is performed which, presumably, depends on the assessor. The acceleration will also depend on the mass of the segment and stiffness of the joint, which can make the assessment difficult in adolescents and adults. Studies of reliability (Fosang et al. 2003; Gracies et al. 2010) differ somewhat but suggest that it is probably best taken as a qualitative indicator of spasticity rather than a quantitative measure. There have recently been several attempts to instrument similar tests using inertial sensors to measure angles and angular velocity (van den Noort et al. 2009)

---

[1] It should be noted that the second definition proposed in this paper is simply a specific form of the first.

Table 8.2 Modified Ashworth Scale modified for measurement of tone

Grade	Description
0	No increase in muscle tone (normal tone)
1	Slight increase in muscle tone, manifested by a catch and release or by minimal resistance at the end of the range of motion when the affected part(s) is moved in flexion and extension
1+	Slight increase in muscle tone, manifested by a catch, followed by minimal resistance throughout the remainder (less than half the range of movement)
2	More marked increase in muscle tone through most of the range of movement, but affected part still easily moved
3	Considerable increase in muscle tone, passive movement difficult
4	Affected part(s) rigid in flexion or extension

Bohannon and Smith (1987).

or electromyography to record muscle activity (van den Noort et al. 2010), but these have not yet been shown to be feasible within a routine gait analysis setting.

There are few systematic approaches to specifying selective motor control at a muscle or muscle group level. The 3-point scale (0/1/2) selectivity described in the section on muscle strength above is probably the only such scale that is widely used in gait analysis. The confusion test (whether dorsiflexion occurs with hip flexion during sitting as part of a flexor synergy) is clearly specific to the dorsiflexors but is sometimes taken as a broader indication of selective motor control and the selective motor control test (Boyd and Graham 1999) is a development of this. The Selective Control Assessment of the Lower Extremity (Fowler et al. 2009) is another recent attempt to try and quantify general selective motor control.

Tests in supine lying

The description of tests below assumes a basic understanding of a conventional physical examination and in particular of muscle length and muscle strength tests. They are described in an order that gives an efficient examination.

Leg Length

Leg length is measured from the ASIS to the distal tip of the ipsilateral medial malleolus, with the patient lying in a supine position. If the patient has a knee flexion contracture, then this should be measured in two segments – from ASIS to medial epicondyle and then from medial epicondyle to medial malleolus. Some centres will also measure the apparent leg length from navel to the medial malleolus.

Hamstrings length

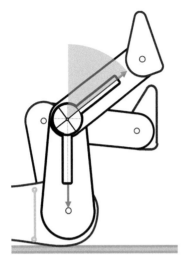

Structures:	Hamstrings.
Position:	Supine, with femur vertical.
Stabilisation:	Flex both hips until ASIS lies vertically over PSIS and maintain position of contralateral femur. The ipsilateral femur is brought back to the vertical (Figure 8.2).
Procedure:	The knee is extended with a sustained stretch until the pelvis starts to move.
Proximal arm:	From lateral epicondyle to centre of ankle joint in sagittal plane.
Distal arm:	From lateral condyle to greater trochanter.
Measure:	Angle from anatomical position. Flexion is positive.

Figure 8.2 Hamstrings length.

This is probably best referred to as the *modified popliteal angle* (Thompson et al. 2001). If the contralateral thigh is lowered to the couch, then the equivalent measure is the *conventional popliteal angle*. The difference between the two has been called the *hamstring shift* (Gage et al. 2009) and arises if a contralateral hip flexion contracture causes an anterior tilt of pelvis away from its standardised position as the thigh is lowered to the couch. The movement of the hamstring origin is such as to limit the range of knee extension available. Hamstring shift is therefore a rather indirect measure of contralateral hip flexor tightness.

Hamstrings spasticity

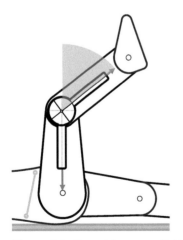

Structures:	Hamstrings.
Position:	Supine, with femur vertical.
Stabilisation:	Opposite limb rests on couch.
Procedure:	Three rapid knee extensions are performed, with the knee held at the angle of catch the third time (Figure 8.3).
Proximal arm:	From lateral epicondyle to the centre of ankle joint in sagittal plane.
Distal arm:	From lateral condyle to greater trochanter.
Measure:	Angle from anatomical position. Flexion is positive.

Figure 8.3 Hamstrings spasticity.

This test is more consistent with the gait analysis data if it is performed with the position of the pelvis standardised as in the previous test. This position makes it difficult for the analyst to perform the test and for the patient to relax, and it is much more common to allow the contralateral thigh to rest on the bed. In this case, measuring the conventional popliteal angle can be useful for comparing the effects of muscle length and spasticity.

Knee extension

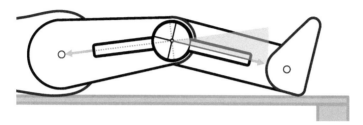

Figure 8.4 Knee extension (flexion as illustrated is negative).

Structures:	Joint capsule and deformity of distal femur or proximal tibia
Position:	Supine.
Procedure:	Knee is extended to end of range, which is generally well defined. Gentle pressure should be applied on the distal femur with counter-pressure under the heel to extend the knee fully (Figure 8.4).
Proximal arm:	From lateral epicondyle to greater trochanter.
Distal arm:	From lateral epicondyle to mid-point of ankle joint in sagittal plane.
Measure:	Angle from anatomical position. Extension is positive.

The lateral malleolus does not provide an indication of the centre of the ankle joint if there is significant tibial torsion and therefore should not be used.

Soleus length

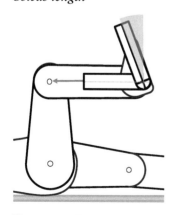

Figure 8.5 Soleus length.

Structures:	Soleus.
Position:	Supine with hip and knee flexed to 90°.
Procedure:	Dorsiflex ankle performing a firm stretch. The mid-foot should be held in sufficient inversion to prevent collapse of subtalar joint (Figure 8.5).
Proximal arm:	From centre of ankle joint in sagittal plane to the fibular head.
Distal arm:	Parallel to lateral border of the plantar surface of hind foot.
Measure:	Angle from anatomical position. Dorsiflexion is positive.

Gastrocnemius length

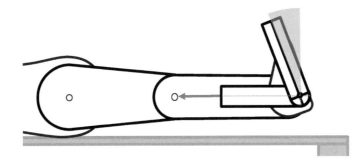

Figure 8.6 Gastrocnemius length.

Structures:	Gastrocnemius.
Position:	Supine with hip and knee extended.
Procedure:	Dorsiflex ankle performing a firm stretch. The mid-foot should be held in sufficient inversion to prevent collapse of subtalar joint (Figure 8.6).
Proximal arm:	From centre of ankle joint in sagittal plane to the fibular head.
Distal arm:	Parallel to lateral border of the plantar surface of hind foot.
Measure:	Angle from anatomical position. Dorsiflexion is positive.

Gastrocnemius spasticity and tone
Gastrocnemius spasticity and tone are also assessed in this position using the modified Tardieu test and modified Ashworth Scale.

Hip abductor length

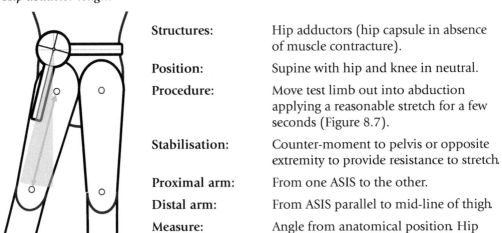

Structures:	Hip adductors (hip capsule in absence of muscle contracture).
Position:	Supine with hip and knee in neutral.
Procedure:	Move test limb out into abduction applying a reasonable stretch for a few seconds (Figure 8.7).
Stabilisation:	Counter-moment to pelvis or opposite extremity to provide resistance to stretch.
Proximal arm:	From one ASIS to the other.
Distal arm:	From ASIS parallel to mid-line of thigh.
Measure:	Angle from anatomical position. Hip abduction is positive.

Figure 8.7 Hip abductor length.

Performing the test over the side of the bed can accommodate a knee flexion deformity. It also allows knee flexion to be used to assess whether any of the hamstrings (particularly gracilis) may be restricting abduction – if so, then repeating the test with the knee flexed to 90° should result in an increased range of abduction. (Abduction can be assessed with hips and knees flexed to 90°, but this is not a particularly functional position for ambulant individuals.)

Adductor tone
Adductor tone is assessed in supine using the modified Ashworth scale. It is very difficult to move the whole lower extremity quickly, and modified Tardieu tests of the hip muscles are difficult in any but very small children.

Knee valgus/varus

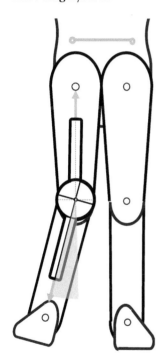

Structures:	Deformity of distal femur or proximal tibia
Position:	Supine in anatomical position. Care is needed to ensure neutral hip rotation particularly if there is any knee flexion contracture (Figure 8.8).
Proximal arm:	From knee joint centre along mid-line of thigh.
Distal arm:	From knee joint centre to ankle joint centre coronal plane.
Measure:	Angle from anatomical position. Valgus is positive, varus is negative. If there is laxity then maximum valgus and range of movement can be recorded.

Figure 8.8 Knee varus/valgus.

This is a modification of the *Q angle* to take into account the whole tibia rather than just its proximal portion. If there is any coronal plane bowing within the tibia, then this should be recorded as it can exaggerate the appearance of varus or valgus on video. Knee valgus is an important measure for quality assurance in gait analysis and should be assessed regardless of whether it is considered clinically relevant.

Hip flexor length

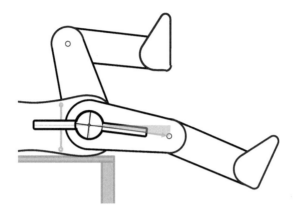

Figure 8.9 Hip flexor length.

Structures:	Iliopsoas (anterior hip capsule in absence of muscle contracture).
Position:	Supine with the buttocks close to the edge of the couch so hip extension is not restricted (Figure 8.9).
Stabilisation:	Flex both hips until ASIS lies vertically over PSIS and maintain the position of contralateral femur.
Procedure:	Allow weight of ipsilateral limb and moderate stretch from examiner to extend hip.
Proximal arm:	Horizontal.
Distal arm:	Long axis of thigh (greater trochanter to lateral epicondyle).
Measure:	Angle from anatomical position. Hip extension is positive.

It is worth checking this test informally after assessing hamstring length. If the hip does not extend beyond neutral, then patient will not have to be moved to the end of the couch. It should be remembered that the weight of the limb places a considerable load on the joint, and if it is not performed over the end of the bed then an equivalent load should be exerted by the examiner.

This *standardised Thomas test* will record about 10° more hip extension than the conventional Thomas test in which the lumbar lordosis is flattened (and the ASIS will be proximal to the PSIS). The use of the standardised test should be clearly indicated when reporting results. The knee should not be too flexed as this may cause the rectus femoris to restrict joint range.

Hip flexor and knee extensor strength
Hip flexor and knee extensor strength can also be assessed while the patient is in the supine position.

Tests in prone lying

Rectus length

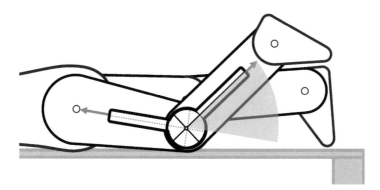

Figure 8.10   Rectus length.

Structures:	Rectus femoris.
Position:	Prone with the hip neutral (or as extended as possible if contractures present) (Figure 8.10).
Procedure:	Flex the knee and apply a reasonable stretch for a few seconds.
Stabilisation:	Pressure should be applied to the buttocks to prevent the hip from flexing.
Proximal arm:	From lateral epicondyle to centre of ankle joint in sagittal plane.
Distal arm:	From lateral condyle to greater trochanter.
Measure:	Angle from anatomical position. Flexion is positive.

A rigorous measurement of rectus length would require standardisation of pelvic position as in the standardised Thomas test which is virtually impossible.

Rectus spasticity

Rectus spasticity is conventionally assessed with the Duncan–Ely test (Bleck 1987; Marks et al. 2003; Kay et al. 2004). The patient is in the same position as for the rectus length test, but the knee is flexed rapidly. The test is considered positive if the patient simultaneously flexes the ipsilateral hip or resistance is felt by the examiner.

Hip internal rotation range

Structures:	Hip joint capsule.
Position:	Prone with hips extended and in neutral rotation and abduction and knees flexed to 90°.
Procedure:	Both hips are simultaneously internally rotated with a reasonable stretch applied (Figure 8.11).

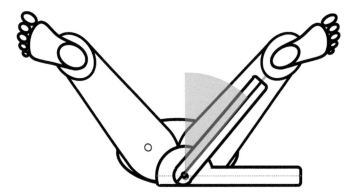

Figure 8.11 Hip internal rotation.

Stabilisation:	Conducting the test bilaterally applies stabilisation but pressure on the buttocks ensures that the pelvis remains horizontal in the transverse plane.
Proximal arm:	Lies on couch.
Distal arm:	Through knee joint centre to ankle joint centre in coronal plane.
Measure:	Angle from vertical. Internal rotation is positive.

All tests of hip rotation and femoral anteversion assume no varus or valgus deformity of the knee. A valgus deformity will bias results to internal rotation (anteversion) and a varus deformity to external rotation (retroversion).

Hip external rotation range
Hip external rotation range can be measured in an equivalent manner but is performed unilaterally (because of the obstruction of other leg if done bilaterally), in which case a counter-moment will be required by placing pressure over the contralateral pelvis to keep the pelvis horizontal in the transverse plane.

Femoral anteversion
Femoral anteversion is also measured unilaterally in this position (Ruwe et al. 1992). The examiner stands on one side of the patient and palpates the greater trochanter on the other side. The examiner then rotates the hip until the greater trochanter is most lateral. This occurs when the femoral neck axis is horizontal, in which position the angle of the tibia from the vertical then specifies anteversion (internal rotation is positive and indicates anteversion, external rotation would indicate retroversion).

Measures of tibial torsion and foot alignment
There are three related measures made with the patient in prone with knees flexed to 90° and the ankles in a neutral position (see Figure 8.12). The examiner must get above the patient to look down on the plantar surface of the foot. The goniometer is not depicted in the figures above for clarity. *Tibial torsion* (left) is the angle between the knee joint

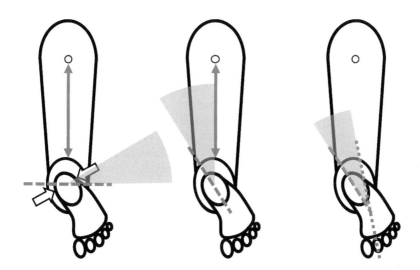

Figure 8.12 Tibial torsion and foot alignment. Refer to text above for detailed descriptions of the three angles depicted.

axis (dashed line, assumed to be perpendicular to the long axis of the femur) and the bimalleolar axis. The two arrows are pointing to the malleoli. The *thigh–hindfoot angle* (middle) is that between the long axis of the femur and the bisector of the heel pad (dashed line). The *hindfoot–forefoot angle* (right) is that between the bisector of the heel pad (dashed line) and the long axis of the forefoot which is assumed to lie along the second ray (dotted line). In the undeformed foot, the hindfoot–forefoot angle will be small. For all measures, external rotation of the distal segment is positive; therefore the shaded angles in the figure for tibial torsion and thigh–hindfoot angle are positive and that for hindfoot–forefoot are negative.

Hip extensor and knee flexor strength
Hip extensor and knee flexor strength can be assessed with the patient in prone, with hips and knees in neutral. Repeating tests of hip extensor strength with the knee flexed may give some indication of the relative strengths of the short and long hip extensors. Ankle plantarflexor strength can be measured in prone with the knees flexed to 90°.

Tests in side lying
Hip abductor strength is the only test performed in side lying. Care is required to ensure that the pelvis is upright in the transverse plane (one hip joint is over the other) in order that hip flexion does not appear as abduction. The body can be stabilised by having the underneath limb flexed at the hip and knee but the pelvis neutral. Ideally both the hip and knee to be tested should be in a neutral position in the sagittal plane. Verbal instruction to lift the leg up towards the ceiling but to also keep the leg back, can be helpful. It may also help the examiner to place his or her arm in front of the patient's

thigh and instruct the patient to avoid touching it by abducting without flexing. Many patients find this test extremely difficult.

Tests in sitting

Dorsiflexor and ankle inverter and everter strength are all assessed in sitting. The *confusion test* (Davids et al. 1993) is positive if active dorsiflexion occurs when the patient is asked to flex the hip against gravity in sitting. Patients with little voluntary control of dorsiflexion are sometimes able to illicit active dorsiflexion in this way. It can be useful to note whether pure dorsiflexion occurs or whether this is accompanied by inversion or eversion of the foot.

Quadriceps lag is the maximum knee extension that the patient can achieve actively and is useful to assess inner range knee extensor function. It is commonly assessed while sitting, although this has the disadvantage that, as the hip is flexed to 90°, the range of movement may be limited by hamstring tightness rather than quadriceps weakness, in which case allowing the patient to lean back a little may help.

Tests in standing

It is useful to assess the posture of the feet in weight-bearing. There are no widely accepted objective scales for this, and a subjective rating of mild, moderate or severe deformity probably represents the state of the art. Recording whether the patient stands in plantigrade is useful. An assessment of whether loading is on the forefoot or distributed over the whole foot would be even more useful but is not possible without instrumentation. The approximate position of the ankle joint in standing should be recorded, bearing in mind that just because the patient is standing on their toes does not necessarily mean that the ankles are plantarflexed. Hindfoot varus or valgus can be recorded as can forefoot abduction or adduction (which may correlate with the hindfoot–forefoot angle recorded in prone lying).

References

Bleck EE. *Orthopaedic management in cerebral palsy.* Oxford, Mac Keith Press, 1987.

Bohannon RW, Smith MB. Interrater reliability of a modified ashworth scale of muscle spasticity. *Physical Therapy,* 1987, 67:206–207.

Boyd RN, Graham HK Objective measurement of clinical findings in the use of botulinum toxin type A for the management of children with cerebral palsy. *European Journal of Neurology,* 1999, 45:s23–35. DOI: 10.1111/j.1468-1331.1999.tb00031.x

Clarkson HM. *Musculoskeletal assessment: joint range of motion and manual muscle strength.* Philadelphia, Williams and Wilkins, 2000.

Dallmeijer AJ, Baker R, Dodd KJ, Taylor NF. Association between isometric muscle strength and gait joint kinetics in adolescents and young adults with cerebral palsy. *Gait Posture,* 2011, 33:326–332. DOI: 10.1016/j.gaitpost.2010.10.092

Davids JR, Holland WC, Sutherland DH. Significance of the confusion test in cerebral palsy. *J Pediatr Orthop,* 1993, 13:717–721.

Fosang A, Baker R A method for comparing manual muscle strength measurements with joint moments during walking. *Gait Posture*, 2006, 24:406–411. DOI: 10.1016/j.gaitpost.2005.09.015

Fosang AL, Galea MP, McCoy AT, Reddihough DS, Story I. Measures of muscle and joint performance in the lower limb of children with cerebral palsy. *Dev Med Child Neurol*, 2003, 45:664–670.

Fowler EG, Staudt LA, Greenberg MB, Oppenheim WL Selective Control Assessment of the Lower Extremity (SCALE): development, validation, and interrater reliability of a clinical tool for patients with cerebral palsy. *Dev Med Child Neurol*, 2009, 51:607–614. DOI: 10.1111/j.1469-8749.2008.03186.x

Gage JR, Schwartz MH, Koop S, Novacheck T. *The identification and treatment of gait problems in cerebral palsy*. London, Mac Keith Press, 2009.

Gracies JM, Burke K, Cleqq NJ et al. Reliability of the Tardieu Scale for assessing spasticity in children with cerebral palsy. *Arch Phys Med Rehabil*, 2010, 91:421–428. DOI: 10.1016/j.apmr.2009.11.017

Kay RM, Rethlefsen SA, Kelly JP, Wren TAL Predictive value of the Duncan-Ely test in distal rectus femoris transfer. *J Pediatr Orthop*, 2004, 24:59–62.

Keenan WN, Rodda J, Wolfe R, Roberts S, Borton DC, Graham HK The static examination of children and young adults with cerebral palsy in the gait analysis laboratory: technique and observer agreement. *J Pediatr Orthop B*, 2004, 13:1–8.

Kendall H, Kendall F. *Muscles testing and function*. Baltimore, Williams and Wilkins, 1949.

Lance J. Pathophysiology of spasticity and clinical experience with baclofen In: Feldman R, Young R, Koella W (Eds.), *Spasticity: Disordered motor control*. Year Book Medical Publishers, Chicago, 1980, pp. 485–495.

Lunsford BR, Perry J. The standing heel-rise test for ankle plantar flexion: criterion for normal. *Phys Ther*, 1995, 75:694–698.

Malhotra S, Pandyan AD, Day CR, Jones PW, Hermens H. Spasticity, an impairment that is poorly defined and poorly measured. *Clin Rehabil*, 2009, 23:651–658. DOI: 10.1177/0269215508101747

Marks MC, Alexander J, Sutherland DH, Chambers HG. Clinical utility of the Duncan-Ely test for rectus femoris dysfunction during the swing phase of gait. *Dev Med Child Neurol*, 2003, 45:763–768.

McDowell BC, Hewitt V, Nurse A, Weston T, Baker RJ. The variability of goniometric measurements in ambulatory children with spastic cerebral palsy. *Gait Posture*, 2000, 12:114–121.

McGinley JL, Baker R, Wolfe R, Morris ME. The reliability of three-dimensional kinematic gait measurements: a systematic review. *Gait Posture*, 2009, 29:360–369. DOI: 10.1016/S0966-6362(00)00068-0

Medical Research Council. *Aids to the examination of the peripheral nervous system*, 1943.

O'Brien MD. *Aids to the examination of the peripheral nervous system*. W.B. Saunders, 2010.

Paternostro-Sluga T, Grim-Stieger M, Posch M et al. Reliability and validity of the Medical Research Council (MRC) scale and a modified scale for testing muscle strength in patients with radial palsy. *J Rehabil Med*, 2008, 40:665–671. DOI: 10.2340/16501977-0235

Ruwe PA, Gage JR, Ozonoff MB, DeLuca PA Clinical determination of femoral anteversion. A comparison with established techniques. *J Bone Joint Surg Am*, 1992, 74:820–830.

Sanger TD, Chen D, Delgado MR et al. Definition and classification of negative motor signs in childhood. *Pediatrics*, 2006, 118:2159–2167.

Sanger TD, Delgado MR, Gaebler-Spira D et al. Classification and definition of disorders causing hypertonia in childhood. *Pediatrics*, 2003, 111:e89–97.

Tardieu G, Shentoub S, Delarue R [Research on a technic for measurement of spasticity]. *Rev Neurol (Paris)*, 1954, 91:143–144.

Thompson NS, Baker RJ, Cosgrove AP, Saunders JL, Taylor TC. Relevance of the popliteal angle to hamstring length in cerebral palsy crouch gait. *J Pediatr* Orthop, 2001, 21:383–387.

van den Noort JC, Scholtes VA, Harlaar J. Evaluation of clinical spasticity assessment in cerebral palsy using inertial sensors. *Gait Posture*, 2009, 30:138–143. DOI: 10.1016/j.gaitpost.2009.05.011

van den Noort JC, Scholtes VA, Becher JG, Harlaar J. Evaluation of the catch in spasticity assessment in children with cerebral palsy. *Arch Phys Med Rehabil*, 2010, 91:615–623. DOI: 10.1016/j.apmr.2009.12.022

Chapter 9
General measures of walking ability

An important role of many clinical gait analysis services is to monitor patients over time. If this is just to record progress without reference to any specific clinical intervention then it is generally referred to as *monitoring*, whereas if it is specifically to assess progress after such an intervention, then it is generally regarded as assessing *outcome*. In whichever context such measurements are taken, the same general principles apply. Whilst any of the measurements described in the earlier chapters can be monitored over time, patients, families and clinicians are likely to be more interested, for these purposes, in general measures of walking ability than in the more technical measures generated during gait analysis or recorded during physical examination. Whilst generally designed to assess progress or outcome, many of these measures are also useful for establishing a context for the interpretation of clinical gait analysis data. Within the Impairment Focused Interpretation framework outlined in the Chapter 12, these measures are most useful in the orientation phase when developing an understanding of who the patient is and why he or she has been referred for clinical gait analysis.

Statistically significant change
Monitoring progress is essentially about establishing whether change has occurred or not. In doing so, it is important to distinguish between statistically and clinically significant changes. Statistically significant changes are those that we can be confident reflect real changes rather than being a consequence of measurement variability. Because many of the measures made during clinical gait analysis have a reasonably high measurement variability, it is particularly important to understand how to determine statistically significant changes. Fortunately this has been a mature science now for nearly a century and is governed by clear and robust principles. It is essential for anyone involved in clinical gait analysis to have a good understanding of these. A full treatment is beyond the scope of this book but some of the key issues are outlined below.

Many people become aware of outcome measures through their use in clinical research. It is important to recognise that measures suitable for assessing outcomes within a group of people in a research context are not necessarily useful for monitoring the progress of individuals. How useful a measure is for assessing change in an individual is fundamentally related to the standard error of measurement (SEM, described in Chapter 13), and this should be stated for any measure being used for monitoring purposes. In order to have 95% confidence that the difference between sequential measurements is real (and not just a consequence of measurement variability), the difference has to exceed 2.8 ($1.96 \times \sqrt{2}$) times the SEM. This is defined as the minimal detectable difference (Portney and Watkins 2009). It is also important to remember that most SEM values have been obtained in carefully conducted research studies incorporating meticulous adherence to measurement protocols. True values for routine clinical practice may be considerably higher. It is therefore extremely important, if such measures are to be used to monitor progress, that the highest possible standards are adopted for making measurements.

Confidence in results can be improved by making repeat measurements. Taking the average of two independent measurements effectively reduces the SEM by a factor of 1.4 ($\sqrt{2}$), but care is needed to ensure that these are genuinely independent measurements. It is very easy for a clinician making a repeat measurement to be biased by the results of the original measure made a short time earlier. Ensuring that repeat measurements are made by the same analyst can also increase confidence that differences between measurements are real. The SEM for measurements made by different analysts will always be greater than that for measurements made by the same analyst (and in many studies the reported SEM is that for different analysts).

In clinical research, the issues are different. The certainty with which the mean value for a group is known is determined by the *standard error of the mean*. Although this sounds similar to the SEM, it is a different quantity and is related to the standard deviation (σ) of all measurements performed on the group. The standard deviation includes variability associated with measurement (characterised by the SEM) and variability between individuals within the group and is therefore always bigger than the SEM. The standard error of the mean, however, decreases with sample size $\left(= \frac{\sigma}{\sqrt{n}} \right)$, and therefore whatever variability there is within and between individuals, the mean value for the group can be measured to arbitrary precision simply by increasing the number of individuals in the group. Measures that have too big an SEM to be useful in monitoring progress in individuals may therefore still have value in comparing performance between groups.

Another particularly important consideration in clinical gait analysis relates to the performance of multiple tests. Requiring that repeat measurements differ by more than 2.8 times the SEM (as described above) only means that this will be indicative of real change on 95% of occasions. If repeat measurements are made of 20 variables, one of them (5% of 20) will be expected to exceed this difference on the basis of the measurement variability alone. Given that gait analysis generates so many variables, this can be expected to occur reasonably often. Whilst techniques for protecting against the risk of false-positives in group analysis are well established they are less well understood in the context of change scores for individuals. Any formal technique for doing so is associated with the risk of missing real change. On balance the best approach is probably to include consideration of the possibility of such occurrences in the subjective interpretation of the data.

Clinically significant change

A clinically significant change is one that makes a difference to the patient. This is inherently subjective but is made even more so as it is generally clinical researchers or clinicians who are the ones devising the measures on behalf of patients. It is best characterised by the *minimal clinical important difference* (MCID), which is the smallest magnitude of change that can be considered important. Methods for determining the MCID are much less well developed than those for statistical significance (Jaeschke et al. 1989; Crosby et al. 2003; Gatchel et al. 2010). Formal definition of an MCID has only been attempted for very few measures in gait analysis (Baker et al. 2012). For more technical measures, it is probably appropriate for clinicians to determine the MCID informally, and they will generally have a good subjective feel for this. Even here, however, the MCID will depend on context. A one-degree change in joint range, for example, may not have any immediate clinical consequences, but if it is indicative of a gradual deterioration which is likely to continue over a long period then it may still be deemed clinically significant. For more general measures it is important to consider the patient's perspective, and formal methods for establishing the MCID are likely to be of more use.

It is particularly important to note that there is not necessarily any correlation between MCID and SEM. Measurements with a small SEM can give real evidence of changes that are of no consequence to the patient. Equally measurements with a large SEM might not give statistical evidence of changes, which have had a marked effect on the patient. In gait analysis measurement variability is generally sufficiently large in relation to MCID that many clinically important changes will be suggested by measurements rather than established conclusively by them. (This is, of course, similar in many fields of contemporary medicine.) This brings an element of subjectivity into the identification and interpretation of change within individual patients.

Classification systems

Classification systems aim to divide people with a certain condition into a number of categories. Generally speaking, such classification is on the basis of characteristics of the condition which are considered unlikely to change. The Gross Motor Function Classification System (GMFCS) divides children with cerebral palsy into one of five functional levels (Palisano et al. 1997, 2008). The definition of these levels varies with age as it is assumed that, as they develop, children in the different levels will achieve different levels of function at different ages. There is growing evidence from longitudinal studies of Canadian children that this is the case (Rosenbaum et al. 2002; Hanna et al. 2008, 2009), and this is generally borne out by clinical experience elsewhere.

Given that the whole point of a classification system is that it differentiates people on the basis of characteristics of a disease or disorder that are assumed to be invariant over time, it does not make sense to use such descriptors as outcome variables. There is a particular issue with many classification systems in that they impose discrete categories on a continuous spectrum of a condition for the convenience of clinicians or clinical researchers. There will always be individuals who are on the border between two levels of the classification. Different clinicians are likely to rate these differently, as may the same clinician rating at different times. More importantly, small variations in the way a borderline person functions as a result of treatment may cause them to appear to rise or fall a level over time. Care should be taken not to overinterpret such changes when they are observed.

The International Classification of Functioning, Disability and Health

Walking ability can be considered at a number of levels. Perhaps the best way of thinking about these is within the context of the World Health Organization's International Classification of Functioning, Disability and Health (ICF) (WHO 2001). Three levels of human disability and functioning are recognised (see Figure 9.1). *Body structures and functions* are physiological functions of body systems or anatomical parts of the body – problems with these are referred to as *impairments*. *Activity* is the execution of a task by an individual and *participation* is involvement in a life situation. The system acknowledges that these levels are not hierarchical. Therefore

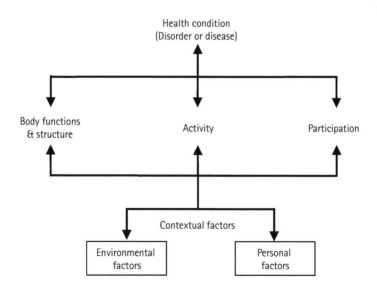

Figure 9.1 International Classification of Functioning, Disability and Health (WHO 2001).

while impairments of body functions often lead to *activity limitations* or *participation restrictions*, those body functions and structures can also be affected by the level of activity and participation. Disability and functioning are viewed as the outcome of interactions between *health conditions* (diseases, disorders and injuries) and *contextual factors*. Those contextual factors can be either external *environmental factors* such as social attitudes, architectural characteristics, legal and social structures, as well as climate and terrain or internal *personal factors* such as sex, age, coping styles, social background, educations and character.

To specify the overall impact of the health condition on an individual, it is necessary to try and quantify the effect at all three levels. This will generally require the use of a range of assessment tools. It is also necessary to assess both *capacity* and *performance*. Capacity indicates a person's ability to perform a task – can they perform a task or not? This is generally directly related to their health condition. Performance indicates whether a person actually does perform a task. This is more obviously a product of both the health condition and contextual factors. Therefore a child may have the capacity to walk around independent of mobility aids but his or her performance may be walking with crutches because (s)he is afraid of losing their balance in a crowded or busy school environment. Most assessments in clinical gait analysis aim to assess a person's capacity to perform tasks.

Walking can be regarded as a physiological function and the gait pattern is specifically listed under the *Neuromusculoskeletal and Movement Related Functions* chapter of the ICF and given the code b770. Most of the general measures of walking ability made during clinical gait analysis also assume walking is a physiological function, and this includes measures of self-selected walking speed, maximum walking speed and energy efficiency. The remainder of this chapter focuses on these.

Walking that occurs as part of everyday life is defined as an activity within the *Mobility* chapter of the ICF. It is further divided into walking over different distances (d4500 and d4501), on different surfaces (d4502) and around obstacles (d4503). For most people, walking will be the main method of moving around the home (d4600), in other buildings (d4601) and for short distances outside the home (d4601). By definition, this activity cannot be measured within the gait laboratory, but questionnaires or data logging devices can be used to obtain the information. This generally does not form part of the clinical gait analysis process, but such measures can be extremely useful to establish the context for interpreting data and are described more briefly below.

Walking ability will also have an effect on how people participate in different life situations. Since the publication of the ICF, various measures focusing specifically on participation have been developed (Noonan et al. 2009; Magasi and Post 2010), but none of these has been used widely in relation to gait analysis. Where broader measures have been used, these have tended to be quality of life tools such as the Short Form-36 (Ware and Sherbourne 1992), Child Health Questionnaire (Landgraf et al. 1996) or Pediatric Outcomes Data Collection Instrument (Daltroy et al. 1998). Although these are all influenced by walking ability, they are not measures of it and will not be covered further in this book.

General measures of walking as a physiological function

Walking speed

Perhaps the most common method for reporting gait speed clinically is to use the speed recorded during the data capture with movement analysis systems. Practice varies somewhat between different services, but this is generally the speed at which the person chooses to walk given no specific instruction and is often referred to as *self-selected walking speed*. Having said this, it is not uncommon for a gait analyst, parent or accompanying health professional to encourage either a faster or a slower walk. Whilst this gives a reasonable indication of walking speed, methods for a more systematic approach to measuring walking speed are probably more appropriate.

Early protocols to measure walking speed were developed as an alternative to measuring oxygen consumption and tended to measure walking speed over relatively long periods (12minutes) presumably because these sort of times are required to obtain reliable oxygen consumption measures to compare them to (Cooper 1968; McGavin et al. 1976). Ten- (Corry et al. 1996; Boyd et al. 1999) and 6-minute (Schwartz et al. 2006) walking tests, measuring oxygen consumption simultaneously with walking speed, have been used for children with cerebral palsy. More recent work has shown that if walking speed is taken as a measure in its own right then shorter times can be used. Butland et al. (1982) showed that 2- and 6-minute tests gave essentially the same results as 12-minute test. In 2002, the American Thoracic Society issued comprehensive guidelines for the administration of a 6-minute walk test (6MWT) which have become standard particularly in respiratory medicine (ATS 2002). A number of studies, however, suggest that a 2-minute tests works just as well for a number of different conditions (Kosak and Smith 2005; Leung et al. 2006; Gijbels et al. 2012). More recently, the validity and reliability of a 1-minute walk test (1MWT) has been established for children with bilateral cerebral palsy (McDowell et al. 2005, 2009; Kerr et al. 2007).

Protocols for all these tests are essentially similar with a 5- or 10-minute seated rest prior to the test followed by an instruction to walk up and down a measured corridor or round a measured track for the given time as fast as possible without running. (It should be noted that this is quite different to the self-selected walking speed that tends to be adopted for gait analysis.) Measurements are generally recorded to the nearest metre. The 6-minute walking distance is undoubtedly most widely used and those applying it in respiratory medicine argue that a shorter test may be a less sensitive measure of respiratory function. Where walking is limited by factors other than respiratory function the shorter tests may be equally informative and clearly take less time.

Timed up and go test

The timed up and go or TUG test (Podsiadlo and Richardson 1991) is widely used in elderly populations as a measure of functional walking ability. It requires a person to sit in a standardised armchair (seat height 46cm, armrest height 65cm), rise from it, walk forward to a line 3m in front of the chair, turn and return to sit on the chair.

The person wears usual footwear and can use a walking aid but no assistance is given. The test is repeated and the time taken for the second test is recorded. The test is obviously dependent on walking speed but also assesses balance and abilities to turn and manoeuvre out of and into the chair. Although it is the time taken that is recorded, the analyst can also observe how the test is performed and videoing of the test is common. Variants include performing the test whilst performing a cognitive (e.g. counting backwards in threes) or manual task (e.g. carrying a glass of water). The American Geriatrics Society, the British Geriatrics Society (2001) and the Society of Nordic Geriatricians (Sletvold et al. 1996) recommend it as a tool for screening for risk of falls.

Gait indices

The Gillette Gait Index (GGI) (Schutte et al. 2000) was the first attempt to define a single figure to describe the quality of the gait pattern. It is a measure of how different a patient's gait is to the mean gait pattern for healthy individuals calculated from 16 univariate gait parameters that were considered by the developers to capture the important features of the gait pattern. The technique required a principal component analysis of data from 71 patients and 24 controls. The index represents the mean square of the distance between a patient's data and the mean data for controls after transforming to the bases of the principal components and scaling to the standard deviation of the reference data. It has a mean value of 15.7, with high values reflecting more abnormal gait patterns.

Although other measures had been proposed (Laassel et al. 1992; Loslever et al. 1994; Tingley et al. 2002; Barton et al. 2007; Chester et al. 2007), the GGI has been most widely cited and validated (Tervo et al. 2002; Romei et al. 2004, 2007; Hillman et al. 2007; Wren et al. 2007; McMulkin and MacWilliams 2008). It has limitations though. The choice of 16 parameters appears arbitrary and mixes temporal-spatial parameters with gait variables. There is no physical meaning to the multivariate components. Tools for calculating the index are not widely available and results appear sensitive to the choice of control data (McMulkin and MacWilliams 2008). The choice of mean square (rather than root mean square, RMS) exaggerates values for more abnormal gait patterns.

The gait deviation index (GDI) (Schwartz and Rozumalski 2008) was developed to address these limitations. It uses data from across the gait cycle for the nine joint angles that are generally regarded as most clinically significant in gait analysis (pelvis and hip angles in three planes, knee and ankle angles in the sagittal plane and foot progression). Data from each side of the 3356 people who had attended gait analysis over a 13-year period were subject to a single value decomposition to identify *gait features*. The first 15 of these were used to form the basis for calculating the RMS distance from the mean values from a reference sample of 166 typically developing children. The resulting measure was not normally distributed. Its logarithm was thus taken and scaled such that the mean value for the control population was 100, and every 10 units below this represent one standard deviation from this mean. The resulting measure showed a good correlation with the GGI (or $ln\left(\sqrt{GGI}\right)$ to be more precise), but significant spread suggests that the two are measures of different aspects of gait pathology. The GDI was found to be normally distributed across people within different levels of the Functional Assessment Questionnaire (see below) and mean values for the different levels were similar increments apart. GDI-kinetic (Rozumalski and Schwartz 2011) uses essentially the same methods to calculate an index based on the kinetic variables. The GDI has now been applied successfully to patients with a range of different conditions including cerebral palsy in children (Rose et al. 2010; Cimolin et al. 2011) and adults (Maanum et al. 2012), amputees (Kark et al. 2012) and children with muscular dystrophies (Sienko et al. 2010).

More recently, Baker et al. proposed the gait profile score (Baker et al. 2009) as the direct RMS distance between an individual's data and the mean normal data calculated across the gait cycle for the same nine joint angles of one side. The resulting measure is normally distributed for the control population (mean 5.3°, standard deviation 1.4°). The distribution of patient data categorised either by GMFCS (for children with cerebral palsy) or by Functional Assessment Questionnaire (FAQ) (all patients) is not normal but its log transform is.

The primary advantage of the GPS is that equivalent measures for the individual kinematic variables can be calculated to give gait variable scores (GVSs), and these can be presented as a bar chart (the movement analysis profile, MAP, see Figure 9.2), which allows an overview of which gait variables are most abnormal. Different combinations of variables can also be used to create other scores such as a sagittal plane score or a hip score. An overall GPS combining hip, knee and ankle variables from both sides, but only one set of pelvic variables, is useful for analyses at the level of the individual person (mean 5.6°, standard deviation 1.4°). Because the score is derived from the control database alone, it is easier to calculate equivalent scores for different gait models (both GDI and GPS are based on the outputs of the conventional gait model) than the GDI which required a large database of people with a range of pathologies. Three studies have developed an equivalent of the GPS for upper extremity movement (Jaspers et al. 2011; Riad et al. 2011; Butler and Rose 2012). The GPS and GVS have been showed to correlate with clinician's subjective opinions of gait data (Beynon et al. 2010) and another study (Baker et al. 2012) has established that the MCID for the GPS is 1.6° representing the difference between adjacent levels of the FAQ. The score has been used to evaluate the outcomes of surgery of children with cerebral palsy (Rutz et al. 2011; Thomason et al. 2011) and to characterise amputee gait (Kark et al. 2012).

The GPS shows a very strong nonlinear correlation with the GDI ($r = 0.995$), and subsequent analysis showed a close mathematical relationship between the GPS and the unscaled GDI (Baker et al. 2009). There is therefore little point reporting both GPS and GDI for the same data. Choice between the two rests primarily on whether a scaled or unscaled score is preferred and whether reference to the MAP enhances interpretation of results.

Energy of walking
A variety of systems are now available to measure oxygen uptake while walking. These can be used to measure respiratory function, which generally requires measurements

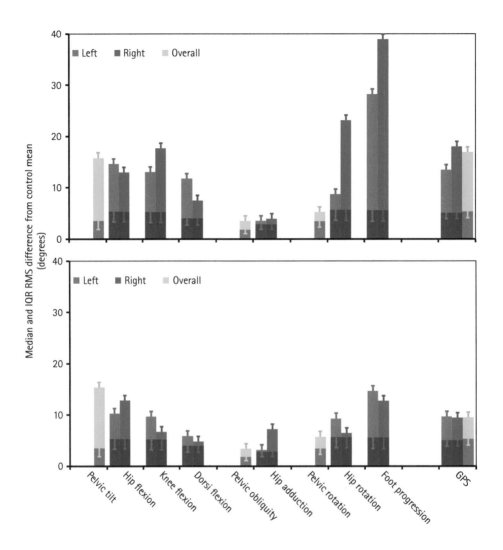

Figure 9.2 Movement analysis profiles (MAPs) for a girl with cerebral palsy before (top) and after (bottom) single event multi-level surgery. Pure colours represent median and interquartile range for the child, darker areas represent equivalent data for healthy controls. The overall global positioning system (GPS) reduces from 16.9° to 9.5°. There have been large changes in the transverse plane, smaller changes at the knee and ankle in the sagittal plane and even smaller changes at the pelvis and hip in the sagittal and transverse planes. Data for the 'left' and 'right' pelvis should be identical so only one is plotted.

of maximal oxygen consumption during some intentionally stressful activity such as fast walking or running. In the context of clinical gait analysis, however, they are used as a measure of the energy cost of walking, most commonly at a person's self-selected walking speed. It is important to remember that these are quite different aims and require quite different methodologies. This book focuses on the latter.

Two measures are generally cited. Oxygen *rate* refers to the oxygen consumed within a given time (*consumption* is also sometimes used in this context in the literature but is also used more generically, so will be avoided). Oxygen *cost* is that consumed in travelling a given distance (typically a metre). Because oxygen is taken as a measure of the energy expended during walking, measures are sometimes converted to Joules per second or per metre. The precise conversion factor depends on the type of food being oxidised within the body, but a value 20.1J/ml O_2 is common (Brockway 1987; Schwartz et al. 2006). Cost can be calculated by dividing the rate (which is the directly measured variable) by the walking speed.

A range of different protocols have been proposed for measuring oxygen uptake. Oxygen rate fluctuates markedly over periods of a few breaths, and an average reading has to be calculated over a reasonable period of time (6–10minutes). Oxygen rate also takes some time to respond to changes in activity level; so the activity needs to be sustained for a period before measurements are made. Some protocols define criteria by which a steady state is recognised and others simply specify a time by which it is assumed to have been attained. Rate can also be affected by a range of factors unrelated to walking ability such as general anxiety levels, and precautions are generally taken to try to standardise test conditions as much as possible. Most protocols therefore also include a period of several minutes rest (3–10minutes) before the walk. Some also specify a period of rest after the test, although there are few reports of how data captured during this period should be used.

There is still some debate over how the data should be normalised. The total oxygen consumed during walking is comprised of the rate measured during rest, which is associated with basic metabolism, and that required for movement. It seems sensible, therefore, to subtract the resting rate from the walking rate to obtain the energy cost of movement. Applying nondimensional normalisation for leg length and weight appears to remove the systematic dependence of the resulting measure on height, weight and age for both rate and cost (Schwartz et al. 2006). It has been suggested that using net rather than gross consumption increases the coefficient of variation for repeat measures in the able-bodied (Thomas et al. 2009a), but the observed increase can be almost entirely attributed to the decrease in the mean value of measurements which results from the subtraction of the resting rate. Essentially the same group of authors, in a paper published in the same year, concluded that net nondimensional cost is the best normalisation method for patient data (Thomas et al. 2009b).

As has been stated in Chapter 2, normalisation is not always appropriate. In particular, it can mask the effects of obesity. An overweight person will take more energy to walk a given distance than a person of normal weight using the same gait pattern but because the values are divided by body mass there may be no appreciable difference in energy consumption. Losing weight will reduce the total energy requirement of movement in direct proportion to the percentage weight loss, but this will not be apparent in the normalised data.

Measures of walking as an activity

Functional assessment questionnaire

The FAQ (Novacheck et al. 2000) records how people walk in real-life situations. It was designed for use in children with cerebral palsy and intended to be completed by a parent. It may be useful more widely. The first part is a list of 10 levels of walking ability, from which the one that best describes the child's typical walking ability is chosen (see Table 9.1).

A second section lists a 22-item skill set, ranging from *walk up and down stairs using a railing*, through *walk carrying a fragile object or glass of liquid* to *ice skate or roller skate*. Parents are asked to select from *easy, little hard, very hard, can't do it at all* or *too young for*

Table 9.1 Levels of the functional assessment questionnaire

1	Cannot take any steps at all
2	Can do some stepping on his/her own with the help of another person. Does not take full weight on feet; does not walk on a routine basis
3	Walks for exercise in therapy and less than typical household distances. Usually requires assistance from another person
4	Walks for household distances, but makes slow progress. Does not use walking at home as a preferred mobility (primarily walks in therapy)
5	Walks more than 15–50 feet (5–17m) but only inside at home or school (walks for household distances)
6	Walks for more than 15–50 feet (5–17m) outside the home, but usually uses a wheelchair or stroller for community distances ot in congested areas
7	Walks outside the home for community distances but only on level surfaces (cannot perform curbs, uneven terrain or stairs without assistance from another person)
8	Walks outside the home for community distances, is able to perform curbs and uneven terrain in addition to level surfaces, but usually requires minimal assistance of supervision for safety
9	Walks outside the home for community distances, easily gets around on level ground, curbs and uneven terrain but has difficulty or requires minimal assistance with running, climbing and or stairs
10	Walks, runs and climbs on level and uneven terrain without difficulty or assistance

Novacheck et al. (2000).

activity. This has recently been subjected to a factor and Rasch analysis, which suggested that the skill set 'is a hierarchical set of interval scales items suitable for measuring locomotor ability in children' (Gorton et al. 2011).

Functional mobility scale
The Functional Mobility Scale (Graham et al. 2004) is similar to the FAQ in that it provides a quick summary of walking status that offers a useful background for interpretation. It is essentially a measure of dependence on walking aids (see Table 9.2) and records this over three different distances: 5m which is taken to represent movement within a room at home, 50m representing movements around a school environment and 500m representing movement within the community.

Activity monitoring
A variety of different devices can be used to monitor walking. There is considerable daily variation in such measures but devices which allow monitoring over several days are now available and in common use. A good way to use these in association with gait analysis is to issue the person with a monitor with a device on the day of the analysis and ask them to post it back to the service on completion of the monitoring period.

Pedometers simply measure step count. More complex devices can also record how step frequency changes over the day. Accuracy can be better than 1% in laboratory conditions (Crouter et al. 2003) but drops with walking speed or when monitoring outside the laboratory (Schneider et al. 2004). As many as 74% of steps have been missed in studies on more marginal walkers (Cyarto et al. 2004). More complex devices based around accelerometers or other inertial sensors can augment simple step count and cadence

Table 9.2 Levels of the functional mobility scale

1	Uses wheelchair, stroller or buggy: May stand for transfers and may do some stepping supported by another person or using a walker/frame
2	Uses K-Walker or other walking frame: without help from another person
3	Uses two crutches: without help from another person
4	Uses one crutch or two sticks: without help from another person
5	Independent on level surfaces: does not use walking aids or need help from another person. If uses furniture, walls, fences, shop fronts for support please use 4 as the appropriate description
6	Independent on all surfaces: does not use any walking aids or need any help from another person when walking, running, climbing and climbing stairs

Graham et al. (2004).

measurements with estimates of step length and hence walking speed. Again such devices perform well in measuring straight-line walking in the able-bodied but are much less effective in real-life situations particularly in patients whose gait pattern may differ from those on which the signal processing is based (Kuo et al. 2009). Systems based on the GPS (Maddison and Ni Mhurchu 2009) are now available but are limited to outdoor use only.

References

American Geriatrics Society. Guideline for the prevention of falls in older persons. American Geriatrics Society, British Geriatrics Society, and American Academy of Orthopaedic Surgeons Panel on Falls Prevention. *J Am Geriatr Soc*, 2001, 49:664–672.

ATS. ATS statement: guidelines for the six-minute walk test. *Am J Respir Crit Care Med*, 2002, 166:111–117.

Baker R, McGinley JL, Schwartz MH et al. The gait profile score and movement analysis profile. *Gait Posture*, 2009, 30:265–269. DOI: 10.1016/j.gaitpost.2009.05.020

Baker R, McGinley JL, Schwartz MH et al. The minimal clinically important difference for the Gait Profile Score. *Gait Posture*, 2012, 35:612–615. DOI: 10.1016/j.gaitpost.2011.12.008

Barton G, Lisboa P, Lees A, Attfield S. Gait quality assessment using self-organising artificial neural networks. *Gait Posture*, 2007, 25:374–379.

Beynon S, McGinley JL, Dobson F, Baker R. Correlations of the Gait Profile Score and the Movement Analysis Profile relative to clinical judgments. *Gait Posture*, 2010, 32:129–132. DOI: 10.1016/j.gaitpost.2010.01.010

Boyd R, Fatone S, Rodda J et al. High- or low-technology measurements of energy expenditure in clinical gait analysis? *Dev Med Child Neurol*, 1999, 41:676–682.

Brockway JM. Derivation of formulae used to calculate energy expenditure in man. *Hum Nutr – Clin Nutr*, 1987, 41:463–471.

Butland RJ, Pang J, Gross ER, Woodcock AA, Geddes DM. Two-, six-, and 12-minute walking tests in respiratory disease. *Br Med J (Clin Res Ed.)*, 1982, 284:1607–1608. DOI: 10.1136/bmj.284.6329.1607

Butler EE, Rose J. The Pediatric Upper Limb Motion Index and a temporal-spatial logistic regression: quantitative analysis of upper limb movement disorders during the Reach & Grasp Cycle. *J Biomech*, 2012, 45:945–951. DOI: 10.1016/j.jbiomech.2012.01.018

Chester VL, Tingley M, Biden EN. An extended index to quantify normality of gait in children. *Gait Posture*, 2007, 25:549–554. DOI: 10.1016/j.gaitpost.2006.06.004

Cimolin V, Galli M, Vimercati SL, Albertini G. Use of the Gait Deviation Index for the assessment of gastrocnemius fascia lengthening in children with cerebral palsy. *Res Dev Disabil*, 2011, 32:377–381. DOI: 10.1016/j.ridd.2010.10.017

Cooper KH. A means of assessing maximal oxygen intake. Correlation between field and treadmill testing. *JAMA*, 1968, 203:201–204. DOI:10.1001/jama.1968.03140030033008

Corry I, Duffy C, Cosgrave AP, Graham HK. Measurement of oxygen consumption in disabled children by the cosmed K2 portable telemetry system. *Dev Med Child Neur*, 1996, 38:585–593.

Crosby RD, Kolotkin RL, Williams GR. Defining clinically meaningful change in health-related quality of life. *J Clin Epidemiol*, 2003, 56:395–407. DOI: 10.1111/j.1469-8749.1996.tb12123.x

Crouter SE, Schneider PL, Karabulut M, Bassett DR. Validity of 10 electronic pedometers for measuring steps, distance, and energy cost. *Med Sci Sports Exerc*, 2003, 35:1455–1460.

Cyarto EV, Myers AM, Tudor-Locke C. Pedometer accuracy in nursing home and community-dwelling older adults. *Med Sci Sports Exerc*, 2004, 36:205–209. DOI: 10.1249/01.MSS.0000113476.62469.98

Daltroy L, Liang M, Fossel AH, Goldberg MJ. The POSNA pediatric musculoskeletal functional health questionnaire: report on reliability, validity, and sensitivity to change. *J Pediatr Orthop*, 1998, 18:561–571. DOI: 10.1097/00004694-199809000-00001

Gatchel RJ, Lurie JD, Mayer TG. Minimal clinically important difference. *Spine (Phila Pa 1976)*, 2010, 35:1739–1743.

Gijbels D, Dalgas U, Romberg A et al. Which walking capacity tests to use in multiple sclerosis? A multicentre study providing the basis for a core set. *Mult Scler*, 2012, 18:364–371. DOI: 10.1177/1352458511420598

Gorton GE 3rd, Stout JL, Bagley AM, Bevans K, Novacheck T, Tucker CA. Gillette Functional Assessment Questionnaire 22-item skill set: factor and Rasch analyses. *Dev Med Child Neur*, 2011, 53:250–255. DOI: 10.1111/j.1469-8749.2010.03832.x

Graham HK, Harvey A, Morris ME, Baker R, Wolfe R. The Functional Mobility Scale (FMS). *J Pediatr Orthop*, 2004, 24:514–520.

Hanna SE, Bartlett DJ, Rivard LM, Russell DJ. Reference curves for the Gross Motor Function Measure: percentiles for clinical description and tracking over time among children with cerebral palsy. *Phys Ther*, 2008, 88:596–607. DOI: 10.2522/ptj.20070314

Hanna SE, Rosenbaum PL, Bartlett DJ et al. Stability and decline in gross motor function among children and youth with cerebral palsy aged 2 to 21 years. *Dev Med Child Neurol*, 2009, 51:295–302. DOI: 10.1111/j.1469-8749.2008.03196.x

Hillman SJ, Hazlewood ME, Schwartz MH, van der Linden ML, Robb JE. Correlation of the Edinburgh Gait Score with the Gillette Gait Index, the Gillette Functional Assessment Questionnaire, and dimensionless speed. *J Pediatr Orthop*, 2007, 27:7–11. DOI: 10.1097/BPO.0b013e31802b7104

Jaeschke R, Singer J, Guyatt GH. Measurement of health status. Ascertaining the minimal clinically important difference. *Control Clin Trials*, 1989, 10:407–415. DOI: 10.1016/0197-2456(89)90005-6

Jaspers E, Feys H, Bruyninckx H, Klingels K, Molenaers G, Desloovere K. The Arm Profile Score: a new summary index to assess upper limb movement pathology. *Gait Posture*, 2011, 34:227–233. DOI: 10.1016/j.gaitpost.2011.05.003

Kark L, Vickers D, McIntosh A, Simmons A. Use of gait summary measures with lower limb amputees. *Gait Posture*, 2012, 35:238–243. DOI: 10.1016/j.gaitpost.2011.09.013

Kerr C, McDowell BC, Cosgrove A. Oxygen cost versus a 1-minute walk test in a population of children with bilateral spastic cerebral palsy. *J Pediatr Orthop*, 2007, 27:283–287. DOI: 10.1097/BPO.0b013e31803433df

Kosak M, Smith T. Comparison of the 2-, 6-, and 12-minute walk tests in patients with stroke. *J Rehabil Res Dev*, 2005, 42:103–107.

Kuo YL, Culhane KM, Thomason P, Tirosh O, Baker RJ. Measuring distance walked and step count in children with cerebral palsy: an evaluation of two portable activity monitors. *Gait Posture*, 2009, 29:304–310. DOI: 10.1016/j.gaitpost.2008.09.014

Laassel EM, Loslever P, Angue JC. Patterns of relations between lower limb angle excursions during normal gait. *J Biomed Eng*, 1992, 14:313–320. DOI: 10.1016/0141-5425(92)90006-7

Landgraf J, Abetz L, Ware JE. *Child Health Questionnaire user's manual*. The Health Institute, New England Medical Centre, Boston, 1996.

Leung AS, Chan KK, Sykes K, Chan KS. Reliability, validity, and responsiveness of a 2-min walk test to assess exercise capacity of COPD patients. *Chest*, 2006, 130:119–125. DOI: 10.1378/chest.130.1.119

Loslever P, Laassel EM, Angue JC. Combined statistical study of joint angles and ground reaction forces using component and multiple correspondence analysis. *IEEE Trans Biomed Eng*, 1994, 41:1160–1167. DOI: 10.1109/10.335864

Maanum G, Jahnsen R, Stanghelle JK et al. Face and construct validity of the Gait Deviation Index in adults with spastic cerebral palsy. *J Rehabil Med*, 2012, 44:272–275. DOI: 10.2340/16501977-0930

Maddison R, Ni Mhurchu C. Global positioning system: a new opportunity in physical activity measurement. *Int J Behav Nutr Phys Act*, 2009, 6:73. DOI: 10.1186/1479-5868-6-73

Magasi S, Post MW. A comparative review of contemporary participation measures' psychometric properties and content coverage. *Arch Phys Med Rehabil*, 2010, 91:S17–28. DOI: 10.1016/j.apmr.2010.07.011

McDowell BC, Humphreys L, Kerr C, Stevenson M. Test–retest reliability of a 1-min walk test in children with bilateral spastic cerebral palsy (BSCP). *Gait Posture*, 2009, 29:267–269. DOI: 10.1016/j.gaitpost.2008.09.010

McDowell BC, Kerr C, Parks J, Cosgrove AP. Validity of a 1 minute walk test for children with cerebral palsy. *Dev Med Child Neurol*, 2005, 47:744–748. DOI: 10.1017/S0012162205001568

McGavin CR, Gupta SP, McHardy GJ. Twelve-minute walking test for assessing disability in chronic bronchitis. *Br Med J*, 1976, 1:822–823.

McMulkin ML, MacWilliams BA. Intersite variations of the Gillette Gait Index. *Gait Posture*, 2008, 28:483–487. DOI: 10.1016/j.gaitpost.2008.03.002

Noonan VK, Kopec JA, Noreau L, Singer J, Dvorak MF. A review of participation instruments based on the International Classification of Functioning, Disability and Health. *Disabil Rehabil*, 2009, 31:1883–1901. DOI: 10.1080/09638280902846947

Novacheck TF, Stout JL, Tervo R. Reliability and validity of the Gillette Functional Assessment Questionnaire as an outcome measure in children with walking disabilities. *J Pediatr Orthop*, 2000, 20:75–81.

Palisano R, Rosenbaum P, Walter S, Russell D, Wood E, Galuppi B. Development and reliability of a system to classify gross motor function in children with cerebral palsy. *Dev Med Child Neurol*, 1997, 39:214–223.

Palisano RJ, Rosenbaum P, Bartlett D, Livingston MH. Content validity of the expanded and revised Gross Motor Function Classification System. *Dev Med Child Neurol*, 2008, 50:744–750. DOI: 10.1111/j.1469-8749.2008.03089.x

Podsiadlo D, Richardson S. The timed "Up & Go": a test of basic functional mobility for frail elderly persons. *J Am Geriatr Soc*, 1991, 39:142–148.

Portney LG, Watkins MP. Foundations of clinical research: applications to practice. Upper Saddle River, NJ, Prentice-Hall, 2009.

Riad J, Coleman S, Lundh D, Broström E. Arm posture score and arm movement during walking: a comprehensive assessment in spastic hemiplegic cerebral palsy. *Gait Posture*, 2011, 33:48–53. DOI: 10.1016/j.gaitpost.2010.09.022

Romei M, Galli M, Motta F, Schwartz M, Crivellini M. Use of the normalcy index for the evaluation of gait pathology. *Gait Posture*, 2004, 19:85–90. DOI: 10.1016/S0966-6362(03)00017-1

Romei M, Galli M, Motta FF, Schwartz MM, Crivellini MM. Analysis of the correlation between three methods used in the assessment of children with cerebral palsy. *Funct Neurol*, 2007, 22:17–21.

Rose GE, Lightbody KA, Ferguson RG, Walsh JC, Robb JE. Natural history of flexed knee gait in diplegic cerebral palsy evaluated by gait analysis in children who have not had surgery. *Gait Posture*, 2010, 31:351–354. DOI: 10.1016/j.gaitpost.2009.12.006

Rosenbaum PL, Walter SD, Hanna SE et al. Prognosis for gross motor function in cerebral palsy: creation of motor development curves. *JAMA*, 2002, 288:1357–1363. DOI:10.1001/jama.288.11.1357

Rozumalski A, Schwartz MH. The GDI-Kinetic: a new index for quantifying kinetic deviations from normal gait. *Gait Posture*, 2011, 33:730–732. DOI: 10.1016/j.gaitpost.2011.02.014

Rutz E, Baker R, Tirosh O, Romkes J, Haase C, Brunner R. Tibialis anterior tendon shortening in combination with Achilles tendon lengthening in spastic equinus in cerebral palsy. *Gait Posture*, 2011, 33:152–157. DOI: 10.1016/j.gaitpost.2010.11.002

Schneider PL, Crouter SE, Bassett DR. Pedometer measures of free-living physical activity: comparison of 13 models. *Med Sci Sports Exerc*, 2004, 36:331–335. DOI: 10.1249/01.MSS.0000113486.60548.E9

Schutte LM, Narayanan U, Stout JL, Selber P, Gage JR, Schwartz MH. An index for quantifying deviations from normal gait. *Gait Posture*, 2000, 11:25–31.

Schwartz MH, Koop SE, Bourke JL, Baker R. A nondimensional normalization scheme for oxygen utilization data. *Gait Posture*, 2006, 24:14–22. DOI: 10.1016/j.gaitpost.2005.06.014

Schwartz MH, Rozumalski A. The gait deviation index: a new comprehensive index of gait pathology. *Gait Posture*, 2008, 28:351–357. DOI: 10.1016/j.gaitpost.2008.05.001

Sienko Thomas S, Buckon CE, Nicorici BS, Bagley A, McDonald CM, Sussman MD. Classification of the gait patterns of boys with Duchenne muscular dystrophy and their relationship to function. *J Child Neurol*, 2010, 25:1103–1109. DOI: 10.1177/0883073810371002

Sletvold O, Tilvis R, Jonsson A et al. Geriatric work-up in the Nordic countries. The Nordic approach to comprehensive geriatric assessment. *Dan Med Bull*, 1996, 43:350–359.

Tervo RC, Azuma S, Stout J, Novacheck T. Correlation between physical functioning and gait measures in children with cerebral palsy. *Dev Med Child Neur*, 2002, 44:185–190. DOI: 10.1017/S0012162201001918

Thomas SS, Buckon CE, Schwartz MH, Russman BS, Sussman MD, Ajona MD. Variability and minimum detectable change for walking energy efficiency variables in children with cerebral palsy. *Dev Med Child Neurol*, 2009a, 51:615–621. DOI: 10.1111/j.1469-8749.2008.03214.x

Thomas SS, Buckon CE, Schwartz MH, Sussman MD, Ajona MD. Walking energy expenditure in able-bodied individuals: a comparison of common measures of energy efficiency. *Gait Posture*, 2009b, 29:592–596. DOI: 10.1016/j.gaitpost.2009.01.002

Thomason P, Baker R, Dodd K et al. Single-event multilevel surgery in children with spastic diplegia: a pilot randomized controlled trial. *J Bone Joint Surg – Am*, 2011, 93:451–460. DOI: 10.2106/JBJS.J.00410

Tingley M, Wilson C, Biden E, Knight WR An index to quantify normality of gait in young children *Gait Posture*, 2002, 16:149–158. DOI: 10.1016/S0966-6362(02)00012-7

Ware JE, Jr., Sherbourne CD. The MOS 36-item short-form health survey (SF-36). I. Conceptual framework and item selection *Med Care*, 1992, 30:473–483.

World Health Organization *International Classification of Functioning, Disability and Health*. World Health Organization, Geneva, 2001.

Wren TA, Do KP, Hara R, Dorey FJ, Kay RM, Otsuka NY. Gillette Gait Index as a gait analysis summary measure: comparison with qualitative visual assessments of overall gait. *J Pediatr Orthop*, 2007, 27:765–768. DOI: 10.1097/BPO.0b013e3181558ade

Chapter 10

Relationships between data of different types

As described in the preceding chapters, a clinical gait analysis involves the capture, collation and comparison of data of a large number of types. Kinematic, kinetic and electromyographic data are captured through a variety of measurement systems. A thorough physical examination and standardised clinical video recording almost always complements this, and a clinical history will often have been obtained from the referral letter, previous clinical notes and a conversation with the patient or their family or carers. Understanding the relationships within this complex dataset is important for ensuring the quality of data (Chapter 11) and as a basis for the interpretation and reporting process (Chapter 12). The quality of data is ensured by recognising that within the total dataset are different measurements of related parameters (and occasionally repeat measures of extremely similar parameters using different techniques). These measurements will not necessarily agree, but they should not contradict each other. If a 5° fixed knee flexion deformity is measured on clinical examination, for example, then minimum knee flexion in walking can be any value above this, depending on what other impairments are present. It should not, however, be below this value. There may be good reasons for the disagreement (e.g. the knee moment applied during gait may be considerably greater than that applied during the clinical examination), but further investigation of such contradictions is an important part of the quality assurance process. It is particularly useful if they can be identified while the patient is still in the laboratory as a repeat of a specific aspect of the clinical examination or a review of marker placement can be very useful to identify the reason for the contradiction.

The interpretation process depends on different aspects of the dataset being brought together to give a better understanding of why the patient is walking as they do. In this process, the different data types augment each other. If minimum knee extension agrees with the measured knee flexion deformity in the example above, then it is likely that the knee flexion contracture is a primary limitation on knee extension during walking. If the minimum knee flexion is considerably less, then there must be other factors affecting the knee. There is a widespread misconception that there should be a direct correlation between physical examination measures and gait data, with several research projects having set out to establish this (McMulkin et al. 2000; Thompson et al. 2001; Desloovere et al. 2006). Indeed, if such strong relationships did exist, then there would be little need to perform the gait analysis. If the knee flexion contracture always predicted minimum knee flexion during walking, then there would be no need to use gait analysis to assess this. Rather, a complex relationship between physical examination measures and gait data should be expected, and the biomechanical unravelling of this relationship is the heart of the interpretation process.

An extremely useful framework for considering how the different data relate to each other is to consider ways in which they can be plotted on gait graphs. Most commonly, this requires a consideration of how specific parameters from the physical examination, for example, can be plotted on the conventional gait graphs. A knee flexion contracture, for example, can easily be plotted as a horizontal line on the sagittal knee angle graph. Sometimes it is useful to plot different parameters on gait graphs to facilitate comparison. Plotting segment kinematics rather than joint kinematics, for example, can be extremely useful when comparing video and gait data for quality assurance purposes (see section below, *Relating gait data to clinical video*). The rest of this chapter, therefore, explores relationships between different types of data by considering how they can be represented on the gait graphs.

Understanding fully the relationship between different types of data is extremely complex and requires an understanding of physiology, anatomy, pathology and biomechanics, which is beyond the scope of this book. It is hoped that what is discussed in this chapter will give an overview of such relationships by covering a number of examples. The reader is encouraged to take this further themselves and consider how relationships between other datasets might be explored using similar or novel techniques.

Relating gait data to clinical video
Gait data should explain what you are seeing on video. It should not contradict it. Therefore, if the thigh appears internally rotated with respect to the line of progression on the video, then the gait data should allow you to determine whether this is coming primarily from transverse alignment of the pelvis or of the hip joint. It should not record that thigh is externally rotated. A comparison of video and gait data can therefore be extremely useful for quality assurance purposes.

The correlation between joint kinematics, upon which most clinical interpretation is based, and the video recording is not always straightforward. Understanding how a particular joint angle as represented on the kinematic graphs will appear on video requires an understanding of the alignment of the proximal segment, which in turn may depend on the alignment of the segment above. To understand the data, therefore, the analyst needs to perform a mental calculation of all the joint angles proximal to the segment in question. Another issue is that the joint will almost certainly not lie in a plane perpendicular to the camera, and so there will be out-of-plane effects.

One solution to these problems is to plot the segment kinematics as projections of the segment principal axes onto the laboratory coronal and sagittal planes. Such angles will be referred to as *segment projection angles* and are illustrated for the segments of the conventional gait model in Figure 10.1. The importance of these angles is that they represent the alignment of body segments as they should appear in a pure sagittal or coronal plane video of the patient. Therefore if the patient is seen to get the foot flat in mid-stance on the video, then the sagittal projection of the long axis of the foot should

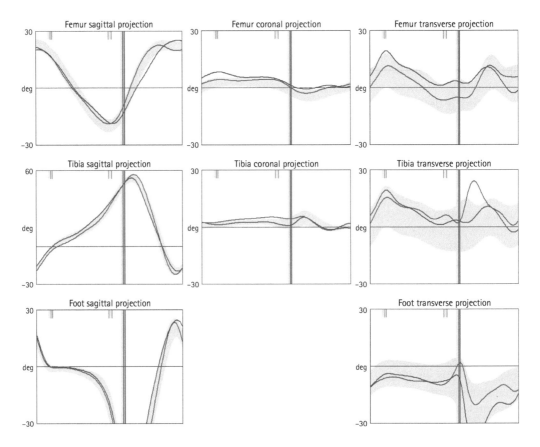

Figure 10.1 Projection angles. The angles between the primary segment and global axes when projected onto the primary global reference planes. These represent the alignment of segments that would be seen on video if the effects of parallax could be removed and are therefore useful for quality assurance purposes. The pelvic kinematics are already quite close to these angles so are not plotted (Fosang and Baker 2006).

be horizontal (0°). If this is not the case, then further investigation of the source of the discrepancy is required. Whilst this technique has been developed as a quality assurance tool, it may also have applications in biomechanical interpretation of the data. Owen (2010), for example, makes substantial reference to segment kinematics in describing the alignment of ankle–foot orthoses. Identification of the four foot rockers as proposed by Perry and Burnfield (2010) also requires reference to the segment as well as to joint kinematics.

Another approach to comparing gait analysis data to the video for quality assurance purposes is to overlay a representation of the model on the video recording. Several manufacturers are introducing this capacity into gait analysis systems. Essentially, a standard video camera is calibrated into the motion capture system that allows joint segments to be added over the video either as line representing joint axes or as meshes representing the bones. If these do not map onto the segments on the video, then further investigation of the problem is required.

One issue with both approaches is that of parallax. This can be minimised by following the principles described in Chapter 7, but it will only be when the patient is in the centre of the field of view and perpendicular to the camera that an exact correlation between segment projection angles and the video should be expected. In theory, parallax effects can be modelled when overlaying segments on the video, but this is rarely convincing in practice. One approach that can be useful is to compare kinematic data with the video for the static pose. The patient is generally stationary in a standardised position in the centre of the field of view. As most errors in marker placement result in fixed offsets in kinematic data (see Chapter 11), checking data from the static trial should increase confidence in those from walking trials. Some care is needed to ensure that the two datasets (video and kinematics) relate to the same static trial – there can be considerable variability in how people choose to stand and they may shift through various postures if asked to stand continuously for some time.

Relating gait data to the physical examination
Whilst the comparison of gait data and clinical video is probably most useful for quality assurance purposes, that between gait data and physical examination data has a much more central role in the interpretation of gait analysis data. As in Chapter 8, this will be described in terms of the different types of tests incorporated in the physical examination.

Bone and joint deformity
Leg length, and particularly relative leg length, is one of the most straightforward measures of bony deformity. If the legs are of different lengths, then this would be expected to be reflected in the degree of pelvic obliquity observed. The natural assumption that the pelvis should be higher on the side of the longer limb, however, is often not the case and may directly reflect other impairments or give insight into compensatory mechanisms. In order to progress beyond a qualitative assessment of such effects, it is necessary to be able to convert from the angular measures that record pelvic orientation (obliquity in particular)

to linear measures of leg length. This will clearly depend on the size of the pelvis, but using Harrington's regression equations (Harrington et al. 2007) it is possible to estimate the distance between the hip joints as a function of the measured inter-anterior superior iliac spine (ASIS) distance (pelvic width). This leads to a simple geometrical relationship between the pelvic obliquity and the difference in hip height,[1] which is represented in Figure 10.2. Thus, if a patient has a pelvic width of 200mm and a measured obliquity of 20°, then one hip will be approximately 50mm higher than the other. This can be compared with the measured leg length discrepancy to understand the extent to which the obliquity can be attributed to this impairment.

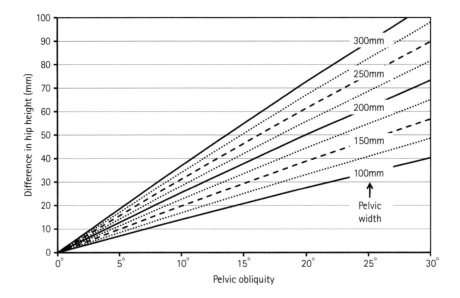

Figure 10.2 Estimated difference in hip height as a function of pelvic width (ASIS to ASIS distance) and obliquity. The same graph can be used to calculate how far one hip is in front of the other for a given degree of pelvic rotation and can therefore be used to estimate the increase in step length that can be attributed to pelvic rotation (which is generally much smaller than is often assumed). ASIS, anterior superior iliac spine.

Measures of torsional deformations of the long bones are also important particularly for the analysis of children with cerebral palsy. Conventionally anteversion is considered as the angle of the femoral neck axis when the knee joint axis is fixed (Figure 10.3, top row), but for gait analysis it is generally useful to think of this the other way round as the angle of the knee joint axis when the femoral neck is fixed (Figure 10.3, bottom row). This is the

---

[1] This is exactly true if the Cardan sequence rotation-obliquity-tilt is used for calculating pelvic angles but only approximately true if other sequences are used (Baker 2001).

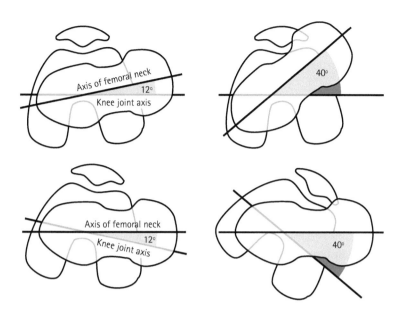

Figure 10.3 Femoral anteversion considered as the position of the femoral neck axis when the knee joint axis is held constant (top) or as that of the knee joint axis when the femoral neck is held fixed. Left-hand side illustrates typical value for an adult (12°) and right-hand side a higher value (40°).

basis of the clinical test for anteversion (Ruwe et al. 1992) in which the femur is rotated until the greater trochanter is most lateral at which point the alignment of the tibia (with the knee flexed by 90°) is used to indicate the degree of anteversion. Femoral anteversion averages about 30° at birth and decreases to about 10° at skeletal maturity except for those with cerebral palsy in which case the higher values of anteversion tend to persist (Bobroff et al. 1999).

The moment arm of the hip abductors is maximised when the femoral neck is close to the coronal plane of the pelvis (Arnold et al. 1997), and if this is the case then the coronal plane of the femur, which is defined by the knee joint axis, will be rotated by approximately the degree of femoral anteversion. Indicating the degree of femoral anteversion on the hip rotation graph can therefore be helpful for interpreting the causes of internal rotation (Figure 10.4). Although the original description of the clinical test for femoral anteversion (Ruwe et al. 1992) recorded excellent agreement with intra-operative measures, it is difficult to perform and is almost always augmented by measures of the range of internal and external hip rotation range, which are measures of the ligamentous constraints on the joint (which can also be plotted along with kinematic data, Figure 10.4). In many people, femoral anteversion is found to be approximately half-way between the limits of internal and external rotations, but it should be remembered that there is no particular reason for this to be taken as a general

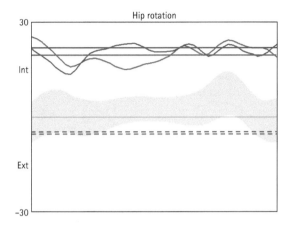

Figure 10.4 Plotting femoral anteversion (solid horizontal lines) and the limit of hip external rotation (dashed horizontal lines) on the hip rotation graph to help with clinical interpretation. The limit of internal rotation could also be plotted but is beyond the range plotted. This suggests that the patient is walking in such a fashion that internal hip rotation is close to the measured femoral anteversion.

principle. It may be particularly misleading after derotation osteotomy when limitations of joint range of movement may be observed over a shorter timescale than can be accounted for by recurrence of the bony deformity.

Tibial torsion is conceptually similar to femoral anteversion, being defined as the angle between the knee joint axis (the coronal plane of the femur) and ankle joint axis projected onto the transverse plane of the tibia. Knee rotation is that of the tibial segment around the long axis of the tibia and, given that the tibial segment is defined by the ankle joint axis, will reflect any true transverse plane rotation at the knee joint *and* the tibial torsion.[2] Plotting tibial torsion on this graph in the same way that anteversion has been plotted in Figure 10.4 is potentially extremely useful. Some software allows tibial torsion to be defined as being equal to the knee rotation measured during the static test. This can be compared with clinical measures of tibial torsion (see Chapter 8) as a quality check. Agreement is not always good, which may reflect measurement variability associated with either technique. It might also be affected by transverse plane motion of the knee between the flexed position in which tibial torsion is usually measured clinically and the relatively extended position during the static trial. If knee extension is generally associated with external rotation of the tibia with respect to the femur (Piazza and Cavanagh 2000), then tibial torsion measured from kinematics during standing would be expected to be greater than that measured clinically.

---

[2] It should be noted that some software such as Plug-In Gait from VICON subtracts off the tibial torsion from knee rotation such that the variable only reflects motion at the knee joint.

Coronal plane knee deformity (varus or valgus) is often clinically important but is also important for quality assurance purposes. Assuming a stable knee, then the knee adduction measured in walking should be fixed and similar to the knee varus or valgus recorded on clinical examination. As with the measures described above, it can be useful to plot this as a horizontal line on the coronal plane knee graph. As described in Chapter 11, poor definition of the transverse alignment of the femur can result in cross-talk from knee flexion occurring as knee adduction. If knee varus or valgus is present then inspection of the knee adduction curves should be relative to this value rather than zero. A further consideration, which is often ignored, is that a valgus deformity will lead to a bias towards internal rotation in clinical assessment of a range of hip internal or external rotation or anteversion. Clinical gait analysis measures orientation of the primary axis of the tibia, the line from knee joint centre to the ankle joint centre. This takes no account of any bowing *within* the tibia. Physical examination measures of knee varus and valgus to supplement gait analysis should reflect this. Any tibial bowing should also be recorded separately, however, as this may be important when comparing coronal plane video with gait kinematics.

Knee extension as measured as a part of the physical examination is essentially a composite measure of bony deformity in the femur or tibia and capsular contracture (or laxity) and, without radiographs, it is virtually impossible to distinguish between these. It is generally assessed in supine with the hip extended, which should slacken off the bi-articular hamstrings. If assessing in other positions, such as sitting, it is important to ensure that it is not the hamstrings that are affecting joint range. The value can be represented on the knee kinematic graph, giving an indication of whether it is the bone/joint deformity that is limiting knee extension or whether other factors are important (see Figure 10.5).

Muscle length
For uniarticular muscles then, joint angle can be used as a direct indication of muscle length. To visualise the relationship between physical examination and gait analysis for such muscles, the range of passive movement on clinical examination can be plotted as a horizontal line across the gait graph in the same way that knee flexion contracture is plotted in Figure 10.5.

Bi-articular muscles are somewhat more complex, with muscle length depending on the positions of two joints. Direct comparison of physical examination and joint kinematics is not possible, but by converting both measurements to muscle length using the same biomechanical model used to calculate muscle lengths during walking (Chapter 5) similar comparisons can be made. Figures 10.6–10.8 contain charts to allow common physical examination measures for bi-articular muscles to be converted to muscle lengths that are comparable to muscle lengths calculated from joint kinematics.

Comparison of muscle lengths during gait with those from physical examination can then be compared. Figure 10.8 illustrates gastrocnemius lengths derived from passive range of dorsiflexion using Figure 10.7. Measurements of 15° and 10° dorsiflexion with

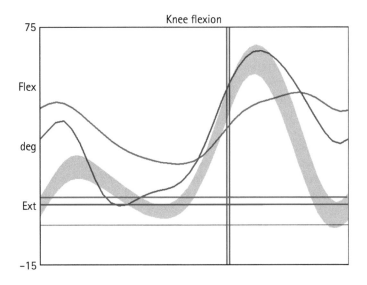

Figure 10.5 Representation of maximum knee extension as measured from physical examination (horizontal lines). On the right side (blue), maximum knee extension in stance is similar to that measured on physical examination, suggesting that it is the knee contracture that is limiting extension. On the left side, the knee does not extend anywhere the limit imposed by the flexion contracture, suggesting other impairments must be limiting extension.

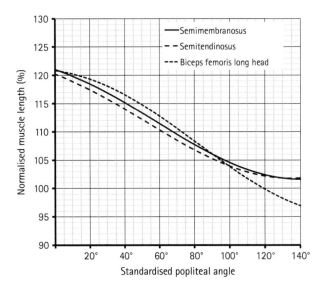

Figure 10.6 Hamstrings muscle length as a function of modified popliteal angle calculated using the same biomechanical model as described in Chapter 5.

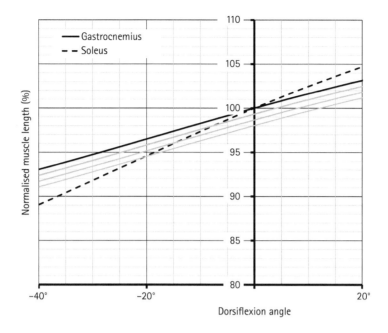

Figure 10.7 Plantarflexor muscle length plotted as a function of dorsiflexion angle and calculated using the same biomechanical model as described in Chapter 5. Grey lines for the gastrocnemius represent knee extension limited by 10°, 20° and 30° knee flexion contractures, respectively, and can be used if full knee extension is not possible during the physical examination.

Figure 10.8 Rectus length as a function of knee flexion with the hip fully extended (0°) calculated using the same biomechanical model as described in Chapter 5.

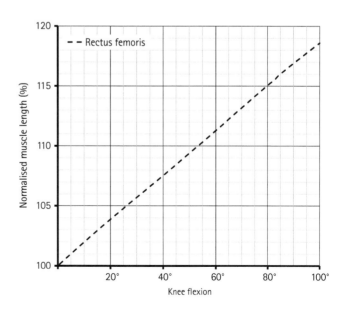

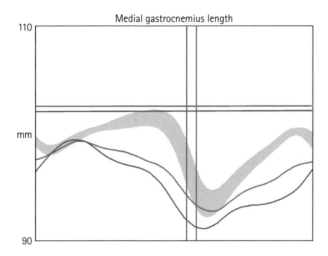

Figure 10.9 Gastrocnemius length from physical examination (horizontal lines) plotted on muscle length graph. See text below <?> for detailed description.

the knee extended equate to muscles lengths of 102.4% and 101.6% respectively. The data show that dorsiflexion during walking appears to be limited by factors other than the gastrocnemius contracture.

Muscle strength
In the same way that PE muscle length measures can be represented on joint kinematic graphs, so quantitative muscle strength measures can be plotted on joint moment graphs. To do this, the moment measured as being generated by the muscle has to be scaled to body dimensions and weight (normalised) in the same way as the joint moments. Fosang and Baker (2006) have presented such data for typically developing children and Dallmeijer et al. (2011) for children with cerebral palsy. This does require dynamometry, standardisation of the location of the dynamometer and either the positioning of the child in such a way that gravity does not affect measurements (Dallmeijer et al. 2011) or that the effect of gravity on measurements is estimated in the modelling (Fosang and Baker 2006). A rather paradoxical finding of such studies is that some patients with weak muscles exhibit higher joint moments than normal during walking. Sometimes there are clear biomechanical explanations for this, but it quite often remains unexplained. Few centres use quantitative measures of muscle strength. Reference to the data of Fosang and Baker (2006) illustrating how grade 5 and grade 3 muscle strength may be useful to consider how qualitative measurements relate to the joint moment graphs.

Neurological signs
Relating neurological signs as identified from physical examination to gait data is particularly challenging. The only test that can be related directly to the gait data is the modified Tardieu test. Given that this measures the catch at a particular angle, then

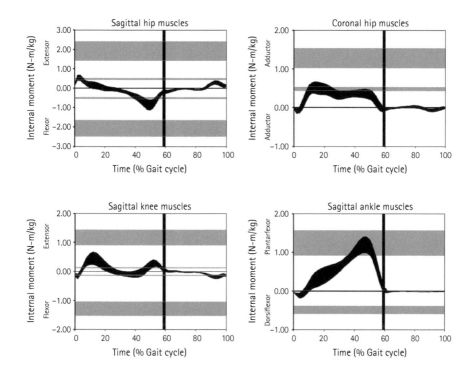

Figure 10.10 Graphical comparison of moment data from walking trials (black) and strength tests (grey). All bands represent the one standard deviation range about the mean calculated from all walking trials or strength tests for all children. The outer (broader) strength bands represent grade 5 strength and the inner (narrower) bands represent grade 3. The grade 3 bands for dorsiflexion and plantarflexion are too close to the horizontal axis to be demarcated (Figure from Fosang and Baker 2006 with permission).

this can be plotted on the gait graphs as with other angles measured during the clinical examination. The test, however, is assumed to be measuring a velocity-dependent response, which happens to occur during the physical examination test at a particular angle. There is no particular reason for such a correspondence between joint angle and joint velocity during walking, which suggests that plotting the modified Tardieu test angle on the kinematic graphs might even be misleading. This is compounded by the fact that the hamstrings, gastrocnemius and rectus femoris muscles to which the Tardieu test is most often applied are all bi-articular muscles and requiring a knowledge of how both joints are moving and not just that at which the measurement was made during physical examination.

There are some features of the gait data that often correlate with high measures of spasticity. It is quite common, for example, to see rapid absorption and then generation of ankle power in first double support. Little work has been done to formally characterise such features, however, and it is therefore difficult to give systematic guidelines as to what to look for in the data A comparison of kinematics during walking and during the static test can also be informative. As spasticity is velocity dependent, it would be expected that patients with neurological signs of spasticity might show greater muscle lengths during standing than during walking. Two studies (Eames et al. 1999; Baker et al. 2002) have used this as a way of quantifying gastrocnemius spasticity and its response to botulinum toxin

In general, however, spasticity is most often identified as an impairment through the absence of direct evidence of other impairments such as muscle contractures or bone or joint deformities. If the neurological signs are positive and there appears no other reason for specific features in the gait data, then attributing them to neurological impairments is sensible.

Relating gait data to electromyography measurements

Muscles cause movement, and there should therefore be a strong correlation between EMG measurements and all gait data This relationship is immensely complex, however, as reflected by research trying to elucidate the role of different muscle during walking (Neptune et al. 2001; Anderson and Pandy 2003; Anderson et al. 2004; Goldberg et al. 2004; Arnold et al. 2005, 2007; Siegel et al. 2006). Muscles act to exert moments around joints, and the immediate effect of these is to cause accelerations. It is only sometime later that this can be observed as changes in joint angular velocities and, even later, in joint angles. When relating EMG to kinematics, it is thus important to remember that changes in kinematics will occur sometime after activity is recorded in specific muscles. The effect on kinematics of activity in a specific muscle will also depend on the activity of other muscles and the alignment and velocities of the limb segments. All of these will be reflected in the magnitude and direction of the ground reaction It is therefore unlikely that a simple relationship will be observed between EMG data and kinematic data The one exception to this is where muscles are overactive for considerable parts of the gait cycle in such a way that they resist movement at particular joints. Examples of this would be overactivity in the rectus femoris, leading to a reduced rate of knee flexion in late stance and early swing or overactivity in the plantarflexors reducing dorsiflexion through stance.

Relationships between muscle activity and gait data should be much more apparent in kinetic data The joint moments calculated using inverse dynamics represent the net moment exerted about the joint by the soft tissues. Ligaments are generally only capable of exerting such moments at the end of joint range (which can be detected by observing how joint kinematics relate to physical examination measures of joint range), and therefore within the range of motion of the joint the moment can be taken as a measure of the net muscle moment. The actual moment generated does not bear a simple relationship to the recorded EMG activity depending on muscle morphology, composition, muscle length, muscle contraction velocity, but the broad pattern of phasic activity should map onto the measured joint moments. In doing so, the possibility of antagonistic activity has to be considered as it is only the net moment that is measured by the joint moment. As mentioned in Chapter 6, EMG activity is much more variable

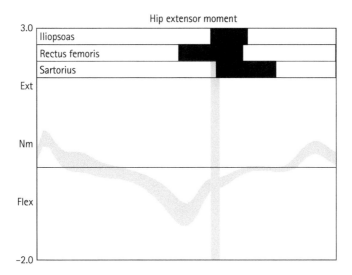

Figure 10.11 Normal hip moment data with timing of EMG activity in muscles that have the potential to act as hip flexors (Lieber 1992) to illustrate how these muscles appear to be active after the late stance hip flexor moment calculated by inverse dynamics.

from cycle to cycle than joint kinematics or kinetics; so this also has to be taken into account. Having said all this, measured EMG activity does not map onto the measured joint moments anywhere near as closely as might be expected, even for normal walking. The most obvious example of this is that hip flexor activity is recorded much too late in the gait cycle to correspond to hip flexor moment as calculated using inverse dynamics (see Figure 10.11). The correspondence between EMG activity and joint moments would benefit from further practical research particularly in the light of the computational studies referred to at the start of this section. Clinical video should not be overlooked in assessing the quality of EMG recordings. Changes in muscle bulk or tendon definition for the major muscles can often be observed from video and should clearly correspond to EMG activation patterns.

References

Anderson FC, Pandy MG. Individual muscle contributions to support in normal walking. *Gait Posture*, 2003, 17:159–169.

Anderson FC, Goldberg SR, Pandy MG, Delp SL Contributions of muscle forces and toe-off kinematics to peak knee flexion during the swing phase of normal gait: an induced position analysis. *J Biomech*, 2004, 37:731–737.

Arnold AS, Anderson FC, Pandy MG, Delp SL Muscular contributions to hip and knee extension during the single limb stance phase of normal gait: a framework for investigating the causes of crouch gait. *J Biomech*, 2005, 38:2181–2189. DOI: 10.1016/j.jbiomech.2004.09.036

Arnold AS, Komattu AV, Delp SL Internal rotation gait: a compensatory mechanism to restore abduction capacity decreased by bone deformity. *Dev Med Child Neurol*, 1997, 39:40–44.

Arnold AS, Schwartz MH, Thelen DG, Delp SL. Contributions of muscles to terminal-swing knee motions vary with walking speed. *J Biomech*, 2007, 40:3660–3671. DOI: 10.1016/j.jbiomech.2007.06.006

Baker R Pelvic angles: a mathematically rigorous definition which is consistent with a conventional clinical understanding of the terms. *Gait Posture*, 2001, 13:1–6. DOI: 10.1016/S0966-6362(00)00083-7

Baker R, Jasinski M, Maciag-Tymecka et al. Botulinum toxin treatment of spasticity in diplegic cerebral palsy: a randomized, double-blind, placebo-controlled, dose-ranging study. *Dev Med Child Neurol*, 2002, 44:666–675.

Bobroff ED, Chambers HG, Sartoris DJ, Wyatt MP, Sutherland DH. Femoral anteversion and neck-shaft angle in children with cerebral palsy. *Clin Orthop Rel Res*, 1999, 364:194–204.

Dallmeijer AJ, Baker R, Dodd KJ, Taylor NF. Association between isometric muscle strength and gait joint kinetics in adolescents and young adults with cerebral palsy. *Gait Posture*, 2011, 33:326–332. DOI: 10.1016/j.gaitpost.2010.10.092

Desloovere K, Molenaers G, Feys H, Huenaerts C, Callewaert B, Van de Walle P. Do dynamic and static clinical measurements correlate with gait analysis parameters in children with cerebral palsy? *Gait Posture*, 2006, 24:302–313. DOI: 10.1016/j.gaitpost.2005.10.008

Eames NWA, Baker R, Hill N, Graham K, Taylor T, Cosgrove A The effect of botulinum toxin A on gastrocnemius length: magnitude and duration of response. *Dev Med Child Neurol*, 1999, 41:226–232.

Fosang A, Baker R A method for comparing manual muscle strength measurements with joint moments during walking. *Gait Posture*, 2006, 24:406–411. DOI: 10.1016/j.gaitpost.2005.09.015

Goldberg SR, Anderson FC, Pandy MG, Delp SL Muscles that influence knee flexion velocity in double support: implications for stiff-knee gait. *J Biomech*, 2004, 37:1189–1196.

Harrington ME, Zavatsky AB, Lawson SE, Yuan Z, Theologis TN. Prediction of the hip joint centre in adults, children, and patients with cerebral palsy based on magnetic resonance imaging. *J Biomech*, 2007, 40:595–602. DOI: 10.1016/j.jbiomech.2006.02.003

Lieber R *Skeletal muscle structure and function: Implications for rehabilitation and sports medicine.* Baltimore, Williams and Wilkins, 1992.

McMulkin ML, Gulliford JJ, Williamson RV, Ferquson RL Correlation of static to dynamic measures of lower extremity range of motion in cerebral palsy and control populations. *J Pediatr Orthop*, 2000, 20:366–369.

Neptune RR, Kautz SA, Zajac FE. Contributions of the individual ankle plantar flexors to support, forward progression and swing initiation during walking. *J Biomech*, 2001, 34:1387–1398. DOI:10.1016/S0021-9290(01)00105-1

Owen E. The importance of being earnest about shank and thigh kinematics especially when using ankle–foot orthoses. *Prosthet Orthot Int*, 2010, 34:254–269. DOI: 10.3109/03093646.2010.485597

Perry J, Burnfield JM. *Gait analysis: normal and pathological function.* Pomona, California, Slack, 2010.

Piazza SJ, Cavanagh PR Measurement of the screw-home motion of the knee is sensitive to errors in axis alignment. *J Biomech*, 2004, 33:1029–1034.

Ruwe PA, Gage JR, Ozonoff MB, DeLuca PA Clinical determination of femoral anteversion A comparison with established techniques. *J Bone Joint Surg, Am*, 1992, 74:820–830.

Siegel KL, Kepple TM, Stanhope SJ Using induced accelerations to understand knee stability during gait of individuals with muscle weakness. *Gait Posture*, 2006, 23:435–440. DOI: 10.1016/j.gaitpost.2005.05.007

Thompson NS, Baker RJ, Cosgrove AP, Saunders JL, Taylor TC Relevance of the popliteal angle to hamstring length in cerebral palsy crouch gait. *J Pediatr Orthop*, 2001, 21:383–387.

Chapter 11
Quality assurance

Capturing movement analysis data is a complex process – this book would not be required if it were not. Clinical gait analysis involves data capture in a clinical environment, requiring the analyst to be attentive to the broader needs of the patient as well as to the specific measurement issues. This can be even more challenging when dealing with children and their parents or carers. The quality of the data is, however, paramount. If we cannot have confidence in the data, there is little point performing the gait analysis in the first place.

Over recent years, quality assurance has been associated increasingly with accreditation processes such as that operated in the United Kingdom by the Clinical Movement Analysis Society or in the United States by the Commission for Motion Laboratory Accreditation. Accreditation is granted primarily on the basis of how well processes are documented. Whilst such documentation is important, it needs to be recognised that this is a minimum requirement. Following instructions is not sufficient to guarantee high-quality measurement in clinical gait analysis. High quality will only be delivered by analysts who understand the measurement processes and are able to review their results critically for evidence of artefacts arising from how that measurement process has been implemented for each individual patient. This is the primary reason why analysts are generally employed at fairly senior levels for healthcare professionals.

The main driver for sustained quality assurance is therefore the critical review of each set of captured data. Clinical gait analysis, including information from the medical history, clinical interview, clinical video and physical examination, contains a rich dataset with strong internal linkages. These links have been outlined in the Chapter 10.

Understanding these linkages, exploring how they are represented in the data and being vigilant for inconsistencies between data from different sources are the main tools that drive the quality assurance process. This quality review process should be an explicit and documented part of every patient analysis. Sometime after the data are captured but before the clinical interpretation starts, the data should be reviewed for evidence of measurement artefact or data inconsistencies. Where artefact or inconsistencies are suspected, these should be clearly documented to avoid the potential for inappropriate inclusion in clinical interpretation.

The most useful time for such a review is while the patient is still in the laboratory with the markers in place. If there are inconsistencies between kinematic data and the physical examination or video, for example, then it is important to be able to check marker placement. Following this logic, it may be useful to check data at an even earlier stage, after the first or second walking trials, for example, allowing for the potential to make changes before continuing with data collection. It may also be useful to repeat an element of the physical examination, though this is generally easier once the markers have been removed. There is often a sense of relief at the end of the analysis for both analyst and patient and the immediate reaction is to strip the markers off and allow the patient to leave. Forewarning the patient that there will be a short period at the end of the analysis while data is reviewed before markers are removed can be useful. Even with this, it is difficult to perform a comprehensive review of data at this stage and the analyst should be focusing on the measurement issues that are of most clinical importance for the individual patient. The comprehensive review can be conducted at a later stage.

A prerequisite of such processes is, of course, that the data are actually available. Some clinical gait analysis software is capable of generating gait graphs within a few minutes of data capture. It is not clear why this is not universal and, in the modern world, it should be a minimum requirement of any system being used within the clinical gait analysis services.

Most of the issues on which such a review should focus have been outlined in Chapter 10. The remainder of this chapter focuses on two particularly important areas of quality assurance – an understanding of the consequences of marker misplacement and of errors in force plate measurement. It should be noted that general aspects concerning accuracy and reliability are discussed in Chapter 13 and issues concerning laboratory and equipment set-up and calibration are covered in Chapter 15.

Consequences of marker misplacement

Marker misplacement is one of the most common sources of variability in clinical gait analysis. Knowing how this affects gait data is important for several reasons. The most obvious is that it allows the identification of features in the data that might be a consequence of marker misplacement. If this is the case, then it is possible to consider what the data might have looked like if markers had been placed more appropriately. If marker misplacement is suspected because of one trace, it is particularly important to understand which other traces will be affected at the same time. Finally, a good understanding of the consequences of marker misplacement generally reflects a good understanding of the biomechanical model being used.

These issues are addressed in this chapter by considering how the gait data for one individual with no neuromusculoskeletal pathology are affected when different markers are moved by 5, 10 and 15mm in particular directions. The data were created by collecting data for a single gait cycle and processing using the conventional gait model (CGM) with the markers applied correctly. Direct alignment of the thigh wands (no knee alignment devices [KADs]) was used and a clinical measure of tibial torsion was used to determine the ankle joint axis with respect to the knee joint axis (no medial malleolus marker). Software was then used to move the markers by a known distance in different directions for both static and dynamic trials and the data reprocessed. In all the graphs, the solid trace represents the original data and the dashed and dotted lines the effects of marker misplacement. The original data came from a 1.4m high male. Broadly speaking, the effects will vary inversely with height; so the magnitude of the angular offsets will be smaller for taller people and more pronounced for shorter.

Data generated using a different biomechanical model will be affected differently by marker misplacement. Indeed the use of other variants of the CGM will lead to some differences. Many of the major effects described below will be similar in other commonly used models, but it is important that the analyst develops an understanding of the particular model they are using to know how effects might differ. Whilst the data graphed out below have been generated using software manipulation of marker positions, similar data can be generated by physically moving markers. Results will not be quite as clear as trial-to-trial variability will be present as well as the effects of marker misplacement. Gait analysts are encouraged to compare the results of such exercises for the model used in their own laboratory with their own predictions of what to expect based on their own understanding of the model.

Pelvic markers
As might be expected, the primary consequence of placing one of the anterior superior iliac spine (ASIS) markers too high is that the pelvic obliquity graphs will be offset so that that the side is recorded as being too high (see Figure 11.1). Hip adduction is the orientation on the thigh relative to the pelvis so if the pelvis is recorded as being higher than it really is then the hip will be recorded as being too adducted by the same amount. There will be a smaller effect on pelvic tilt. If one ASIS marker is too high, then this will raise the mid-point between the ASIS markers by half the marker offset, and this will result in a small decrease in anterior pelvic tilt (see Figure 11.2). This in turn will have the effect of recording a mild increase in hip extension. There is no appreciable effect on pelvic rotation.

If the orientation of the pelvis is changed, then the estimated position of the hip joint centres will also change (see Figure 11.2). If the ASIS marker is placed higher, then the ipsilateral hip joint will be higher by almost the same amount. The increased pelvic obliquity has the consequence of moving the estimated hip joint centre a small distance laterally on the ipsilateral side and medially on the contralateral side. These effects are smaller than the direct effects of pelvis position and are therefore masked in the sagittal and coronal planes, but a small effect on hip internal rotation can be observed, which

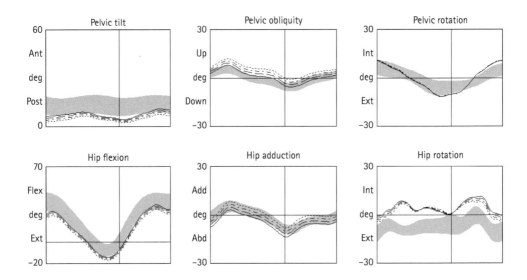

Figure 11.1 The effect of placing an anterior superior iliac spine (ASIS) marker too high. Solid line is original placement, dashed line is 5mm too high, dash–dotted line is 10mm to high and dotted line is 15mm too high. Data from a 1.4m tall person. Effects more distally are minimal.

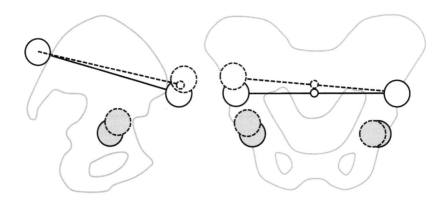

Figure 11.2 The effect on the estimated position of the hip joint centre as a consequence of an anterior superior iliac spine (ASIS) marker being placed too high. Original marker and hip positions are depicted by solid lines, misplaced markers and altered hip joint centres by dashed lines. See text above for explanation.

arises from an interaction between the hip flexion angle and the altered position of the hip joint centre. As the CGM is hierarchical, there is the potential for effects on the knee and ankle graphs, but these are found to be minimal.

Moving an ASIS marker laterally makes very little difference to any of the traces generated using the CGM. The principal axis of the pelvis is defined as passing from one axis to the other; so it is unchanged by displacing either marker along this direction and so is the pelvic orientation. The mid-point between the two ASIS will be shifted towards the laterally displaced marker but only by half the marker displacement. As a consequence, the estimated position of both hip joint centres will move by half the displacement towards the misplaced marker, resulting in increased ipsilateral adduction and decreased contralateral abduction. In practice, the effects are barely discernible on the graphs with about 1° of difference for every 10mm of misplacement.

The posterior superior iliac spine (PSIS) markers are only represented in the model through their mid-point, and then the only effect this has is on pelvic tilt about the line from one ASIS to the other. If both markers are placed too high, then the pelvis will appear more anteriorly tilted (about 3° for every 10mm misplacement) and the hip will therefore appear more flexed. There will be similar but opposite effects on the hip joint locations to those depicted in Figure 11.2, but again these are small in comparison to the direct effects on pelvic alignment. If only one of the PSIS markers is too high, then the effects will be halved because the mid-point of the PSIS markers will only be raised by half the misplacement of one marker. The mediolateral position of the PSIS markers is irrelevant in the CGM and misplacement in this direction will not affect gait traces at all.

Thigh, knee and KAD markers
As the CGM is hierarchical, misplacement of markers below the pelvis can have no effect on the pelvis kinematics. How the thigh and KAD markers affect the data depends on which variant of the CGM is used. Figure 11.3 illustrates the effects of placing the thigh wand marker too far forwards by 5, 10 and 15mm, which for a 50mm long wand represents rotations of approximately 3°, 6° and 9° about the base plate. Very similar graphs will be obtained if the KAD is used and rotated internally by these same angles. Given that the thigh marker is used to define the internal or external rotation of the femur about the line between the hip joint centre and knee marker, it should be no surprise that internal hip rotation increases by the same angle as the thigh wand is anteriorly rotated. Because the tibial segment rotation is defined by the tibial markers (using this variant of the CGM), the internal rotation of the femur will lead to relative external rotation of the knee joint.

An important feature for quality control purposes is that there is also an effect on the knee adduction trace (Kadaba et al. 1990; Baker et al. 1999). To a good approximation, the tibia moves in a single plane with respect to the femur (in the absence of knee joint deformity or laxity). If the thigh marker is placed correctly, then this plane is the same as the sagittal plane of the femur. Large amounts of knee flexion and minimal amounts of knee adduction are generally observed. If the thigh marker is placed too far forwards, however, the sagittal plane of the femur will be internally rotated and knee movement will no longer occur within it. A phenomenon called cross-talk will occur, in which knee flexion will 'appear' as increased knee adduction. This is similar to the effect that occurs if an observer stands in front of a person walking with externally

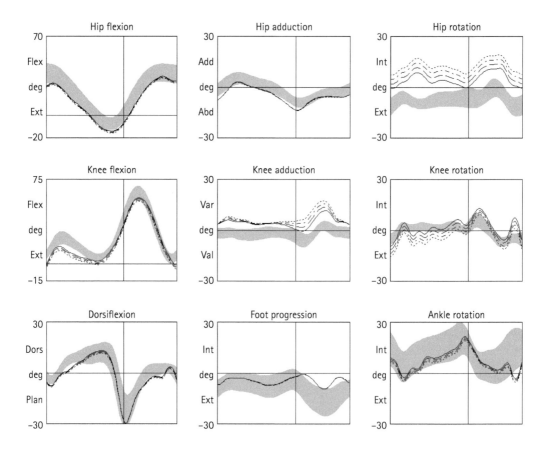

Figure 11.3 The effect of placing a thigh wand marker too anteriorly. The solid line is the original placement, dashed line is 5mm too far forwards, dash–dotted line is 10mm and dotted line is 15mm. Data from a 1.4m tall person.

rotated femurs. As the knee flexes, the person appears to show knee adduction (the opposite effect is more commonly observed when people walking in internal rotation appear to have abducted knees which can be mistaken for knee valgus). Because the knee is most flexed in swing, the increased adduction is most pronounced in swing, and there is sometimes evidence of increased adduction at the peak of stance phase knee flexion as well (see Figure 11.3). The more that the shape of the knee adduction curve looks like that of the knee flexion graph then the more likely it is that the thigh wand has been placed anteriorly. If the wand has been placed too posteriorly, then the opposite effect will cause the knee adduction curve to look like a mirror image of knee flexion in the horizontal axis. This phenomenon can be extremely useful for quality assurance as it gives a clue to when thigh markers (or knee alignment devices) may have been incorrectly placed. Changes to the knee adduction curves are rarely of clinical significance, but the erroneous hip rotation curves that such characteristics indicate are often of considerable importance.

There are certain cases when this technique may not work. If the knee is stiff throughout gait, then there is no sagittal plane movement to generate cross-talk. If the knee is stiff and flexed, then an error in thigh marker placement would be expected to result in a fixed offset on the coronal plane knee graphs. This can be extremely difficult to distinguish from a genuine varus or valgus deformity of the knee. The technique also assumes that there is little true knee adduction; if there is knee laxity then this may not be the case. Because this is such an important technique for quality assurance, it can be useful to assess the knee joints for any laxity or deformity during the physical examination regardless of whether these are considered clinically important or not. In doing this, it is important to remember that the gait analysis system is based on the overall alignment of the femur and tibia between knee joint centre and hip and ankle centres, respectively. Knee angles are not affected by localised deformity in the distal femur or proximal tibia to any greater extent than this has on the overall alignment of the bones.

There is another minor consequence, which is that if the thigh marker is too anterior then the coronal plane of the femur will be internally rotated and the knee joint centre will be estimated as being too posterior (Figure 11.4a). Knee flexion will therefore be underestimated by a small amount. This even has a small effect on the measured ankle dorsiflexion and rotation (see Figure 11.3). Misplacing the marker up or down along the long axis of the thigh will have no effect on the model outputs as the marker is only used to determine rotations about this axis.

The only differences if the KAD is used are in knee and ankle rotation. Use of the KAD effectively sets the knee rotation during the static calibration to zero by rotating the tibia internally by the same angle as the femur. In this case, misplacement does not affect knee rotation at all but the ankle (alignment of the foot with respect to the tibia) will appear externally rotated.

It can be seen from Figure 11.4b that moving the knee marker anteriorly will have an opposite effect to moving the thigh marker anteriorly and result in overestimation of external hip rotation. The rotation of the coronal plane of the knee results in the knee joint centre being estimated as even more anterior than the direct effect of the misplacement, which will lead to overestimation of hip and knee flexion and dorsiflexion.

Tibial and ankle markers
As with the thigh markers, given the hierarchical nature of the CGM, misplacement of markers on the tibia can only affect the kinematics of the knee and more distal joints. Figure 11.5 shows the effects of moving the tibial marker too anteriorly (assuming direct alignment of wand markers is used, i.e. no KAD calibration). It can be seen that misplacing the marker anteriorly introduces an artefactual internal rotation of the tibia segment, which leads to overestimation of knee rotation and underestimation of ankle rotation. There will be similar effects on the ankle joint centre as illustrated in Figure 11.4 for the knee, but because the knee is narrower this has a smaller effect on knee flexion

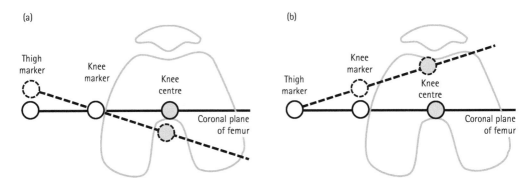

Figure 11.4 Transverse plane view of femur markers to illustrate the effect of thigh (a) and knee (b) marker misplacement on the knee joint centre. Solid lines represent accurate marker placement. Dashed lines represent misplaced markers and the effect on the estimated knee joint centre (grey fill).

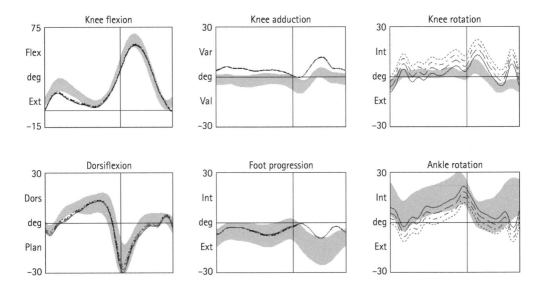

Figure 11.5 The effect of placing a tibial wand marker too anteriorly. The solid line is the original placement, dashed line is 5mm too far forwards, dash–dotted line is 10mm and dotted line is 15mm too far forwards. Data from a 1.4m tall person.

and dorsiflexion. In a number of variants of the CGM (with KAD, or medial malleolar marker or supplying a clinical measure of tibial torsion), then misplacement of the tibial marker will have no effect on model outputs as long as it is in the same place for static calibration and walking trials. The model is insensitive to misplacement of the marker up and down along the long axis of the tibia whichever variant is used.

Misplacing the ankle marker anteriorly will have a similar effect on the ankle to anterior misplacement of the knee marker on the knee (see Figure 11.6). The estimated ankle joint centre will be too anterior, leading to a small underestimation of knee flexion and dorsiflexion.

Foot markers
Changes to the markers on the foot can only affect the ankle and foot graphs. Changes are generally quite predictable. Medial or lateral misplacement of the toe marker will lead to overestimation of internal or external foot progression and ankle rotation. The more proximal the placement of the marker, the more sensitive the model will be to misplacements of a fixed linear distance. Because the line between the heel and toe markers during the static trial is taken as being parallel to the long axis of the foot, medial and lateral movements of the heel marker will have an opposite effect.

Kinetics
Marker misplacement will have an effect on kinetic as well as on kinematic data. Differences will arise both because the estimated position of joint centres may have changed and also because the segment coordinate systems in which the moments are represented may have changed alignment. Effects will depend on whether the proximal or distal segment coordinate system has been used. In this exercise, the proximal segment was selected for all joints.

The effects on kinetic data of marker misplacement are generally less significant than the kinematic effects. Figure 11.7 illustrates the largest change to kinetics generated by varying any of the marker placements. Because the estimated knee joint centre is too anterior (see Figure 11.4), the knee extensor moment is overestimated and there is a smaller effect on total knee power but apart from this the effects are quite minimal.

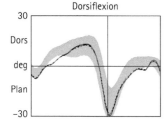
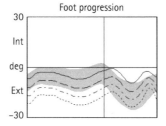
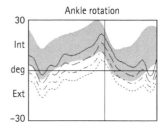

Figure 11.6 The effect of placing a forefoot marker too laterally. The solid line is the original placement, dashed line is 5mm too far forwards, dash–dotted line is 10mm and dotted line is 15mm too far forwards. Data from a 1.4m tall person.

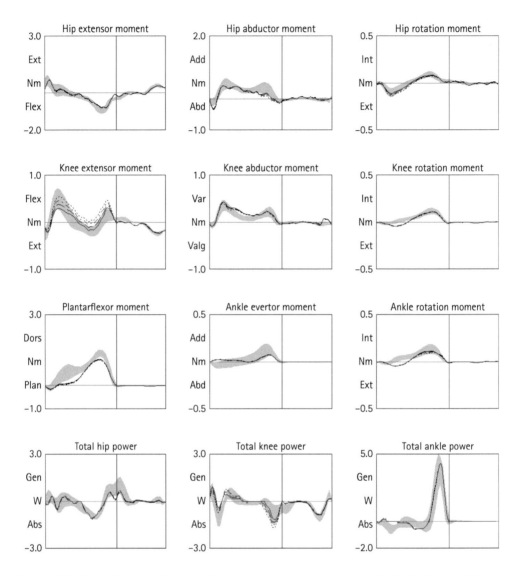

Figure 11.7 The effect on kinetics of placing a knee marker too anteriorly. The solid line is the original placement, dashed line is 5mm too far forwards, dash–dotted line is 10mm and dotted line is 15mm too far forwards. Data from a 1.4m tall person.

Consequences of errors in force plate measurements

There are three probable sources of error from force plates: hardware malfunction, failure to determine location and orientation within the calibration of the kinematic measurement system and failure to correctly identify which foot has contacted the force plates. Methods for protecting against the first two are described fully in Chapter 15,

Setting up a Clinical Gait Analysis Laboratory. Identifying foot contacts is judged visually at the time of capturing data in most centres. To give valid data for the whole of stance phase, a foot must be entirely within the boundaries of the plate for all of this period and no part of the other foot, anyone else's foot or any walking aid should make contact with the plate during that time either. This clearly requires that force plate outlines are visible and that someone is closely watching to judge the steps for which valid force plate data have been collected. If a model requiring a small number of foot markers is being used, then applying additional markers to indicate the outline of the foot can be extremely useful for checking data retrospectively. Placing markers on the heel, tip of hallux and 1st and 5th distal metatarsal heads gives an excellent indication of where the foot has been placed in relation to the plates. These can also be useful to check that the centre of pressure lies within the boundaries of the foot.

Sticks and crutches are often placed laterally and miss the plates. Under these circumstances, joint kinetics are still valid in the sense that they reflect the moments that the internal structures (primarily the muscles) are exerting at the joints. It is, however, important to take stick and crutch use into account when interpreting the results clinically. A reduction in moments should be expected, for example, if bodyweight is shared between the limbs and crutches.

Recognising errors in force plate measurement from kinetic data

The most obvious sources of error in kinetics arise when there are discontinuities in the data These are likely to arise when another part of the body or a walking aid makes contact with a plate but can arise for other reasons as well. The data in Figure 11.8, for example, have arisen because of incorrect zeroing of one of the force plates. It should be remembered that various smoothing filters are applied by the software; so discontinuities of the data as plotted may not be as obvious as might be expected. It is also important to remember that if there is evidence on artefact on one kinetic trace, then it is virtually certain that data at the same point in the gait cycle for all other kinetic traces are likely to be invalid. Errors in kinetic data arising from failure to identify invalid force plate contacts will tend to vary somewhat from trial to trial (as foot placements tend to vary somewhat from trial to trial as well). Therefore individual kinetic traces looking different from the majority of other traces should always be treated with suspicion. Because the mass of the foot is so small, there should never be a significant ankle moment recorded during swing. If there is, then kinetic data for the ankle and hip should also be regarded with suspicion.

Joint moments and powers require integration of force plate measurements with kinematic data and, on the rare occasions that faults do occur, they are not always easy to identify. Plots of the individual ground reaction should always be checked for quality assurance purposes. The moments at the hip, however, are the most sensitive measurements for most potential force plate faults. Even quite small errors in determining the direction of the ground reaction can lead to quite substantial differences in the hip moments. Perhaps equally importantly, many problems that can develop with the force plates will affect the data captured with the patient walking in one direction

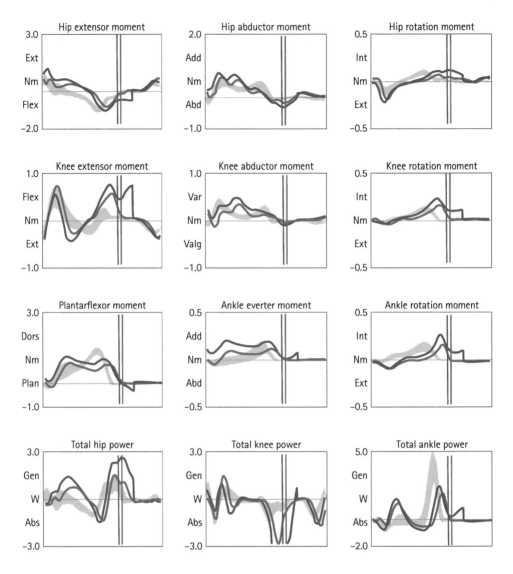

Figure 11.8 Error in force plate data resulting in marked discontinuities on right side in early swing. There are discontinuities in several traces occurring at the same time in the gait cycle.

in the opposite way when they are walking in the opposite direction. Therefore if the gain on the anterior–posterior component of the ground reaction is wrong, it will result in the hip moment to be underestimated when the patient is walking in one direction and overestimated when walking in the other direction. There will be similar issues with coronal plane measurements. If mild, these will increase the apparent variability in hip

Figure 11.9 Hip abductor moment data captured with incorrect force plate location. Five walks in one direction overestimate the moment throughout stance. Moments are underestimated for the four walks in the other direction. Data provided by Julie Stebbins who had intentionally introduced an 20mm error in mediolateral force plate location to illustrate this phenomenon.

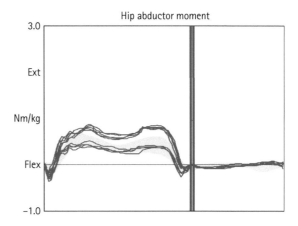

moments (indeed the observation that, generally, moments are reasonably consistent is testimony to the quality of most force plate installations). If more serious, then these can result in two families of traces being present in the data depending on which way the patient was walking (Figure 11.9). Similar effects for measurements from different plates can also be observed if one plate is working correctly but the other has developed a fault. If such stratification is observed, then it is important not only to be wary of data for that particular patient but also to perform checks on equipment (see Chapter 15) to ensure that there is not a fault with the hardware which may affect other patients as well. It should be noted, however, that with the trend for laboratories to use more and more force-plates the effects of any one plate malfunctioning can be much harder to spot.

References

Baker R, Finney L, Orr J. A new approach to determine the hip rotations profile from clinical gait analysis data. *Hum Mov Sci*, 1999, 18:655–667. DOI: 10.1016/S0167-9457(99)00027-5

Kadaba MP, Ramakrishnan HK, Wootten ME. Measurement of lower extremity kinematics during level walking. *J Orthop Res*, 1990, 8:383–392. DOI: 10.1002/jor.1100080310

Chapter 12
Interpretation and reporting

In consultation with Jennifer McGinley, Fiona Dobson and Pam Thomason

The primary output of any analysis should be a report of what that analysis has revealed. Reports of findings can therefore be regarded as the core product of gait analysis services. Despite this, there is little agreement as to what an ideal gait report should look like and how it should be produced. This chapter outlines the basic principles that should be embodied in any interpretation and reporting process and then illustrates how these are embodied within one particular approach, impairment focused interpretation (IFI). This has been developed specifically for the reporting of data collected to assist orthopaedic surgeons in planning complex surgery for children with cerebral palsy.

General principles

Perhaps the most important characteristic of any report is that it should be *relevant*. This requires a consideration of who the report is being written for. In most clinical services, the report is being written for the clinician who has referred the patient. Sometimes that clinician will have specified a particular question that he or she would like answered but, more often than not, there is no well-defined question. Under these circumstances, the assumed aim of the analysis is to describe the factors that are limiting the patient's walking ability. Given this, the report should state these as clearly as possible.

The report also needs to be *succinct*. This is essential to ensure the efficient use of time of both the person reading the report and the person writing it. Whilst being succinct, however, it also has to be *comprehensive*. The gait analyst has a duty of care to ensure that a complete and thorough interpretation of the data communicated to the referring clinician. If interpretation were a purely objective process then reporting results would be sufficient. There are, however, significant subjective elements in the interpretation of most gait analysis data, and this requires the report to be *transparent* in documenting how the conclusions have been reached from the data presented. These steps should be *evidence based* wherever possible.

A final factor is that the report should be written *within the competencies of the authors*. This will, of course, depend on who is involved in the reporting team. A variety of appropriately trained staff may be deemed competent to apply biomechanical principles to gait analysis data to determine what is wrong with the patient. Only those with specific professional backgrounds should offer formal treatment recommendations. Therefore, the only person who should recommend specific orthopaedic surgery for a given child is an orthopaedic surgeon.

In some leading centres, the gait analysis data are interpreted within the context of a broader multi-disciplinary decision-making process. A variety of factors might be discussed including reports from other diagnostic tests, medical imaging, the psychosocial background of the patient and family, local resources and expertises and the preferences of the family and clinicians. All these factors are essential for the clinical decision-making process, but they are not part of the gait analysis. There is a real risk that introducing these into the discussion at too early a stage will lead to a lack of focus and corresponding loss of quality of the gait analysis itself. To protect against this, it is useful to adopt an explicit two-stage process. In the first stage, the gait analysis data are interpreted to give a concise description of why the person is walking the way they do which is recorded in a formal gait report. In the second stage, this information can be integrated with all the other relevant factors to make a clinical decision about what action is to be taken.

Impairment focused interpretation

Definitions
This particular interpretation and reporting technique has evolved specifically for children with cerebral palsy who are being assessed prior to a complex orthopaedic surgery. That surgery aims to remove or reduce the effect of a range of *impairments* that are affecting the child. Each child with cerebral palsy has a different number of such impairments, and the aim of the gait analysis is to identify the specific impairments that are affecting the individual child in order that the orthopaedic surgeon can decide how to proceed. This is achieved by considering *features* in the gait data and relating these to *supplementary data* such as that arising from the physical examination.

The italicised terms in the preceding paragraph are used in a specific sense and require further definition in this context. An *impairment* has already been defined by the World Health Organization as *a problem in body structures or functions such as significant deviation or loss* (WHO 2001). Examples may be at least as useful as this formal definition and, for a child with cerebral palsy, might be such things as hip flexion contracture, gastrocnemius spasticity, persistent femoral anteversion or gluteus medius weakness.

Each of these examples specifies a specific body structure (such as a bone or muscle) and what is wrong with it (which is generally one of spasticity, contracture, deformity or weakness).

A *feature* is a specific aspect of the gait analysis data that is considered clinically significant or, in other words, something that can be seen on one of the graphs. Examples might be increased anterior pelvic tilt throughout the gait cycle, too much right plantarflexion at initial contact, hip rotation within normal limits throughout cycle bilaterally and increased left plantarflexor moment in early stance. In order to describe a feature completely, the side (left, right or bilateral), timing (phase of the gait cycle), the gait variable (pelvic tilt, plantarflexor moment, etc.) and the nature of the feature (too much, too little, too early, too late, etc.) must all be specified.

If a feature is anything that can be seen on one of the graphs, then *supplementary data* refer to any relevant information that is not displayed on the graphs. The most obvious examples are measurements from the physical examination such as limited range of extension of left hip on clinical examination or increased resting tone of plantarflexors bilaterally. Other data that are known at the time of the analysis can also be included such as results from medical imaging.

Orientation

A four-stage process has been developed to support IFI: *orientation, mark-up, grouping* and *reporting*. The first stage, orientation, is to understand the patient's background. The diagnosis should be known including any relevant classifications of the condition such as the topographic distribution and Gross Motor Function Classification System (Palisano et al. 1997, 2008) grading if the child has cerebral palsy. The overall level of motor function should also be recorded through either scales such as the Functional Assessment Questionnaire (Novacheck et al. 2000) or the Functional Mobility Scale (Graham et al. 2004) or general comments. A brief relevant history should include details of previous surgical or other interventions and current medical, physiotherapeutic and orthotic provision. The final component of orientation to the patient is a summary of the reason for referral.

The second stage of orientation is to the walking pattern. Having a broad impression of how the patient was walking during the test session is an important safeguard against misinterpretation of gait data. This starts through visual observation of gait during the test session, which can be important to ensure that the data recorded are representative of the patient's general level of capacity and performance. An important question to be asked of the patient and any family member attending with him or her is whether the gait pattern adopted during the test session is representative of their usual walking pattern. Orientation to the walking pattern also requires a consideration of the temporal spatial parameters. It is important to understand how quickly the patient is walking, how cadence and stride length contribute to this and how much asymmetry there is (primarily reflected in step length). Speed is known to affect gait patterns in typically developing children (Schwartz et al. 2008), and this may be relevant to how the gait data are interpreted.

Orientation to the walking pattern should also include a brief review of video recordings (and brief notes of these may be useful within the report). The use of video alongside three-dimensional gait data is often misunderstood. The three-dimensional data should allow a better understanding of what can be seen on video but should not contradict it. If the patient is walking with the knee facing forwards, for example, the three-dimensional data should record how much of this is a consequence of pelvic rotation and how much of hip rotation. If the three-dimensional data record the knee as facing inwards or outwards, however, in contradiction to the video, then this suggests that there is something wrong with the measurement process. Videos recorded simultaneously with the three-dimensional data are more useful for this purpose as the possibility of discrepancies arising from genuine differences in the way the patient walked between video and three-dimensional recordings is excluded.

The third and final stages of orientation, which leads on from this, is to the data. It is important to look over the data before proceeding with any detailed interpretation to look for any issues that might affect that interpretation. Checking the consistency of data from multiple walks gives an understanding of how variable the gait pattern is and how much importance can be given to any particular feature from one specific walk. Many gait laboratories superimpose data from a number of walks as multiple traces (colour coded for left and right) as the basic format for reporting, which allows consideration of variability to be incorporated throughout the interpretation process. The mark-up stage in IFI can be very messy with multiple traces, however, and may be useful to select a single trial for mark-up.

Historically gait analysts have preferred to analyse a representative trial rather than the mean trial which has advantages and disandvantage. Averaging may smooth out features that are present in the underlying trials but occur at slightly different times. On the other hand the representative trial might contain features that are only present for that trial and are not characteristic of the patient. It is also rare to find a single trial that is representative of the patient for all gait variables. On balance the average trial is probably a safer alternative as a basis for clinical intperpretation and, working within an clincal govenrance framework, this is probably the most important criterion. Whichever is selected a good understanding of the consistency of data for the patient being analysed is an important part of the analysis. (It should be noted that selecting a representative trace in research studies may lead to under-estimating variability in measurements and hence increases the risk of identifying false positive results. In this context random sampling or inclusion of all valid data is generally prefereable.)

Mark-up

Mark-up is the process of marking features on gait graphs using a range of symbols. The exact symbols used are not particularly important, but suggestions are given in Table 12.1. Features exhibited on one side only are marked in the colour used for the traces (red for left and blue for right in this book) and those exhibited bilaterally are marked in a third colour (green in this book). A letter is placed next to each symbol to identify it during grouping.

Table 12.1 Suggested symbols for use during mark-up

↑	Increased (all of cycle)	↓	Decreased (all of cycle)		Arrow ending on trace
⊕	Too much (part of cycle)	⊖	Not enough (part of cycle)		On trace (or just above or below feature)
←	Too early	→	Too late		Arrow ending on feature
←→	Too long	→←	Too short		Arrow spanning feature
⬍	Increased range	⬌	Decreased range		Adjust height and width as appropriate
◿ or		◹	Abnormal slope		Sloping side along feature
✔	Within normal limits				Only use if particular reason for doing so
?	Possible artefact				On feature
◯	Other feature				Encircling feature

Each symbol can be considered to represent four properties that are summarised by the symbol: type (too much, increased range, etc.), side (left, right or bilateral), variable (knee flexion, plantarflexor moment, etc.) and timing (phases of gait cycle). When learning the process of mark-up, it can be useful to complete a table listing the properties each symbol represents but this is not essential once this has been mastered. It is sensible to adopt a systematic approach to mark-up. Starting at the top left-hand kinematic graph and working through the columns in order before moving onto the kinetic data is one such approach. Although not essential, systematic labelling of features can make it easier for someone reading the report to identify them later. There is a particular issue with pelvic traces. There is only one pelvis so the left and right side traces both reflect the single pattern of pelvis movement in different ways. It is therefore generally only necessary to mark features for one side of the pelvis.

There are often several ways to identify any given feature. A 'bump' in a trace, for example, could be identified by the one *too much (part of cycle)* symbol or an *increasing and decreasing slope* symbol on either side. It is not particularly important how any feature is marked up as long as it can be clearly identified during the grouping process. There may also be some variability between whether a particular feature is described as too much of one variable or not enough of its opposite. Feature *b* in Figure 12.1, for example, could be described either *as too much knee flexion* or *not enough knee extension* (see Table 12.2). Which is chosen is not particularly important. Sometimes one of the alternatives will be more clinically appropriate, but often the two are equally appropriate and the choice is arbitrary. How big a feature needs to be before it is marked by a symbol also requires some judgement. Sometimes it might be useful to consider the magnitude of the feature as a fifth property. Much of the variability in how the data are marked up will depend on which features are of most clinical interest for patients with a particular condition. Coronal knee moments, for example, may be seen as clinically more significant for children with spina bifida than for those with cerebral palsy.

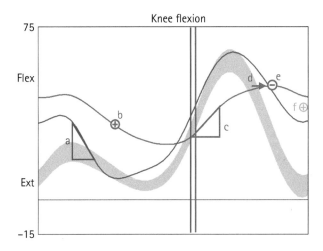

Figure 12.1 Example of mark-up for a knee flexion graph. These are colour coded such that features relating to the left side are marked up in red, for the right in blue and bilateral features are marked up in green.

Table 12.2 Summary of mark-up symbols for Figure 12.1

	Type	Side	Variable	Timing
a	abnormal slope of	right	knee flexion	in early single support
b	too much	left	knee flexion	throughout single support
c	abnormal slope of	left	knee flexion	through foot off
d	too late peak of	left	knee flexion	in swing
e	too little	left	knee flexion	in swing
f	too much	bilateral	knee flexion	at foot contact

Grouping

This stage requires grouping of all features and supplementary data that are considered to be associated with a specific impairment. Therefore in the data presented in Figure 12.2, for example, the bilateral increased anterior tilt (feature *a*) and increased hip flexion (feature *b*) are both commonly associated with contracture of the hip flexors. The supplementary data that are associated with this are the passive ranges of hip extension

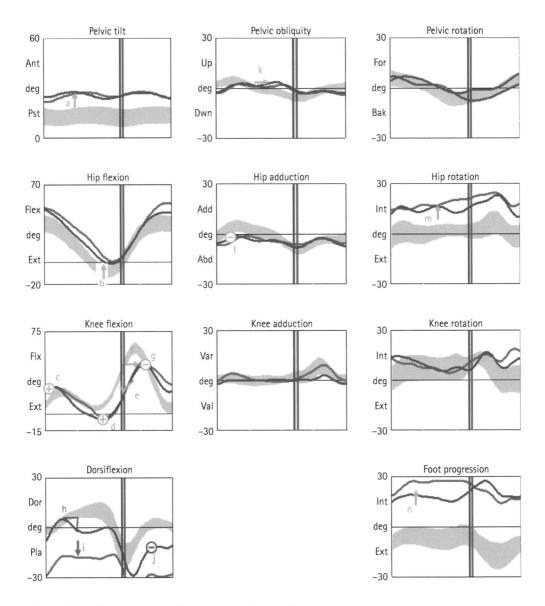

Figure 12.2 Full mark-up of an array of kinematic graphs.

(Thomas test), which in this case are approximately 15° less extension than exhibited by typically developing children. Therefore the group of these two features and one physical examination measure is associated with an impairment of bilateral hip flexion contractures. This group can be summarised in a *grouping box* as illustrated in Figure 12.3 (other grouping boxes for this data are illustrated in Figure 12.4). There is some subjectivity in this process, and it is important to indicate the confidence in the findings. In Figure 12.3, the evidence for this particular impairment is described as *clear* (other options are *probable* and *possible*). It is also useful to have some indication of what impact the impairment is having on the walking pattern. In Figure 12.3, this is described as major (other options are *moderate* and *minor*).

Grouping is a skill that takes some time to learn. Experienced gait analysts develop an ability to identify groups very quickly and efficiently and beginners will take considerably longer. It is important, particularly for less experienced analysts, to develop a flexible approach. When first forming groups they should be considered as provisional and there may be a need to transfer features and supplementary data from one group to another as the analyst develops a fuller understanding of the data (using copy and paste functions within a word processor makes this particularly straightforward). As this process continues, the groups become more refined and definitive.

The clearer the association of features and supplementary data with specific impairments, the more transparent the interpretation will be. Generally speaking, the analyst should attempt to associate each feature or supplementary datum with a different impairment. Achieving this generally reflects a good understanding of the data. There are exceptions, however; an oblique pelvis, for example, could be associated with both a true leg length discrepancy and a functional leg length discrepancy arising as a consequence of a unilateral contracted gastrocnemius. Multiple associations are therefore possible, but should always be reviewed to ensure that they are genuine. The converse is a feature that the analyst cannot associate with a specific impairment. These too are rare but should be listed in the report so that the referring clinician is aware that there are unexplained features within the data.

Impairment: **Bilateral hip flexion contracture**			Evidence: **clear**	Effect on walking: **major**
Features:			Comments:	
a. too much pelvic tilt through cycle				
b. too much bilateral hip flexion through cycle				
Supplementary data:	left	right	Comments:	
Thomas test	5°fl	5°fl	Modified test – TD value 10° ext	

Figure 12.3 Grouping box recording features and supplementary data that indicate an impairment of bilateral hip flexion contracture for the data presented in Figure 12.2.

Impairment: **Bilateral hamstrings contractures**		Evidence: **probable**	Effect on walking: **moderate**

Features:		Comments:	
c. Too much knee flexion at initial contact			

Supplementary data:	left	right	Comments:
Popliteal angle	50°	45°	
True popliteal angle	55°	55°	
Dynamic popliteal (Tardieu)	65°	55°	Dynamic values little higher than true popliteal angle suggesting mostly contracture

Impairment: **Bilateral persistent femoral anteversion**		Evidence: **clear**	Effect on walking: **major**

Features:		Comments:	
m. too much bilateral hip int. rot. through cycle			
n. too much bilateral int. foot prog. through cycle			
l. too little hip adduction in early stance		Wide base of support to allow toes to clear each other.	

Supplementary data:	left	right	Comments:
Hip internal rotation range	90°	90°	
Hip external rotation range	5°	10°	
Femoral anteversion	45°	45°	

Impairment: **Left gastroc and soleus contracture**		Evidence: **clear**	Effect on walking: **major**
Impairment: **Right gastroc contracture and spasticity**		Evidence: **clear**	Effect on walking: **major**

Features:		Comments:	
j. Too much left plantarflexion through cycle			
h. Rapid right plantarflexion in early single support		Sign of spasticity	
i. Too little right dorsiflexion in swing			
d. Too much left knee extension in late stance		Toe walking increases knee flexion moment.	
k. Max pelvic obliquity too late in stance		Knee extension increases leg length through single support.	

Supplementary data:	left	right	Comments:
Dorsiflexion (knee 90°)	10°pf	5°df	
Dorsiflexion (knee 0°)	15°pf	10°pf	
Dynamic dorsiflexion (Tardieu)	25°pf	20°pf	

Impairment: **Bilateral rectus spasticity**		Evidence: **possible**	Effect on walking: **moderate**

Features:		Comments:	
f. Reduced max knee flexion in swing bilaterally		Could be consequence of too much knee extension in late stance.	
g. Max knee flexion too late bilaterally			
e. Slope of knee flexion through toe-off is normal		would expect to be reduced if rectus is spastic	

Supplementary data:	left	right	Comments:
Duncan-Ely slow	none	none	
Duncan-Ely fast	mild	mild	

Figure 12.4 Grouping boxes for other impairments derived from the data illustrated in Figure 12.2.

Reporting

The final stage requires documentation of the interpretation process in a format that it most useful to the referrer. The report needs to start with the basic identification of the patient and the reason they were referred (if this was stated explicitly within the referral letter). Most patients are referred to find out specifically what is wrong with them; so the most important information is the list of impairments that should also appear on the front page. This should be followed by any comments that are considered relevant to clinical decision-making, which might be based on the impairment list. A list of unassociated features, for example, might indicate that the impairment list only represents a partial explanation of the gait pattern. Some patients appear to develop walking patterns that 'use' specific impairments beneficially (e.g. some rely on spasticity to maintain support of bodyweight). If this is the case, then the referrer might need to be warned that interventions aimed at removing that specific impairment might have negative as well as positive consequences. Figure 12.5 therefore illustrates a typical front page for a gait report.

Gait Analysis Report

Patient and referral details					
Name: **Fred Bloggs**			Age: **10yrs 3mths**		
Diagnosis	**CP (diplegia)**	GMFCS	**II**	FMS	**665**

Reason for referral:
Assessment prior to single event multi-level surgery

Findings

The most likely impairments affecting the walking pattern are:

Bilateral hip flexion contracture	Evidence: **clear**	Effect on walking: **major**
Bilateral hamstrings contractures	Evidence: **probable**	Effect on walking: **moderate**
Bilateral persistent femoral anteversion	Evidence: **clear**	Effect on walking: **major**
Left gastroc and soleus contracture	Evidence: **clear**	Effect on walking: **major**
Right gastroc contracture and spasticity	Evidence: **clear**	Effect on walking: **major**
Bilateral rectus spasticity	Evidence: **possible**	Effect on walking: **moderate**

Other comments:
All significant features of the kinematic data have been associated with one of the impairments listed above

Signed

Richard Baker

Prof Richard Baker,
PhD CEng CSci MIPEM,
Clinical Scientist.

Date: 2nd July 2012

Figure 12.5 Front page of an impairment focused gait report.

If gait analysis was an entirely objective and conclusive process, then there would be no need to supply any other information. Because there are subjective elements in the interpretation, it is, however, important to be transparent in describing how the listed impairments have been identified. The report also needs to contain brief details of the orientation process (Figure 12.6) and the grouping boxes for the identified impairments (Figures 12.3 and 12.4). Finally, the report should include a copy of the marked up graphs, the consistency plots and a tabulated summary of the physical examination.

The final report therefore documents the interpretation process but does so in an order suited to the referring clinician. This is different to the order in which the interpretation was performed. This can be facilitated by using a word processor template set out for the final report, with the different sections being filled in as the different stages of interpretation are completed. Therefore graphs and physical examination data are imported first and then the orientation sections are completed. Next the grouping boxes

---

Orientation:

Relevant history:
No previous Botulinum toxin injections or surgery.
Reports increased tripping and difficulty in participating in sport at school.

Height	**1.4m**	Weight	**31kg**	Speed	**80%**
All temporal-spatial parameters normalised to leg length and	Cadence	**101%**	Stride length	**79%**	
expressed as % of those for children with no neuromuscular pathology.	Left step length	**80%**	Right step length	**78%**	

Comments on video:
Generally impression of quite functional gait. Walks on toes bilateral (equines looks worse on left). Knees are flexed at initial contact but extend reasonably well in late stance. Has flexed hips and lumbar lordosis throughout cycle. Both hips appear internally rotated with internal foot progression.

Quality

Is the data likely to be representative of the subject's usual walking pattern?
Yes

Are there any concerns regarding consistency of traces?
Generally quite consistent with a little more variability distally.

Is there any evidence of measurement artefact or inconsistency in the data?
Gait traces suggest mild hyperextension in late stance that is not apparent on video or on physical examination. Marker placement might be biased towards knee extension.

Figure 12.6 Summary of orientation process suitable to include in gait report.

are filled out and finally the impairment list is transcribed onto the cover page. All the information that the referrer needs if he or she is prepared to accept the opinion of the gait analyst at face value is contained on the front page. All the information required to understand how that opinion was derived is contained on the inside pages. A final page gives brief annotation of abbreviations used in reporting the physical examination results and a key to the symbols used in mark-up. Figure 12.7 illustrates a seven-page report covering barefoot kinematics and physical examination. Clearly more inside pages will be required if kinetics and electromyography have been captured and if data from more than one walking condition are available.

Treatment recommendations
If suitably qualified health professionals are included within the gait analysis team, then treatment recommendations can be included with the report. Generally speaking, these should only be made by a health professional who would make treatment decisions if they had responsibility for clinical management of the child. Therefore only an orthopaedic surgeon should make surgical recommendations whereas a physiotherapist or orthotist might make recommendations within their own area of professional

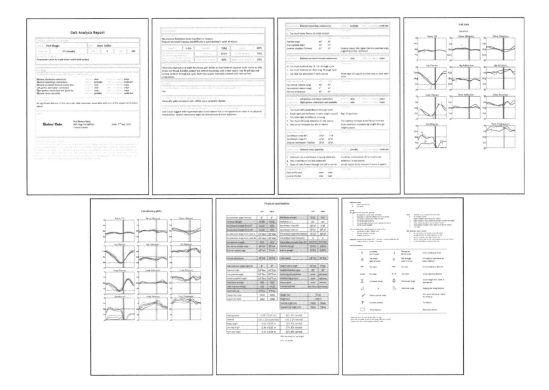

Figure 12.7 A seven-page gait report giving comprehensive documentation of kinematic data for bare foot walking and physical examination.

competence. It should be remembered that treatment decisions are context specific depending on the availability, expertise and experience of relevant health professionals, the availability of access to specialist facilities and the specific preferences of patients and their parents or other carers. It is for this reason that the specification of definitive impairment list does not generally translate directly into unambiguous treatment recommendations. Further guidance on treatment recommendations is regarded as outside the scope of this book, which is intended primarily as a handbook for gait analysts.

References

Graham HK, Harvey A, Rodda J, Nattrass GR, Pirpiris M. The Functional Mobility Scale (FMS). *J Pediatr Orthop*, 2004, 24:514–520.

Novacheck TF, Stout JL, Tervo R. Reliability and validity of the Gillette Functional Assessment Questionnaire as an outcome measure in children with walking disabilities. *J Pediatr Orthop*, 2000, 20:75–81.

Palisano R, Rosenbaum P, Walter S, Russell D, Wood E, Galuppi B. Development and reliability of a system to classify gross motor function in children with cerebral palsy. *Dev Med Child Neurol*, 1997, 39:214–223.

Palisano RJ, Rosenbaum P, Bartlett D, Livingston MH. Content validity of the expanded and revised Gross Motor Function Classification System. *Dev Med Child Neurol*, 2008, 50:744–750. DOI: 10.1111/j.1469-8749.2008.03089.x

Schwartz MH, Rozumalski A, Trost JP. The effect of walking speed on the gait of typically developing children. *J Biomech*, 2008, 41:1639–1650. DOI: 10.1016/j.jbiomech.2008.03.015

World Health Organization. *International Classification of Functioning, Disability and Health*. World Health Organization, 2001.

Chapter 13

Accuracy and measurement variability

In consultation with Jennifer McGinley

Ensuring the quality of the data obtained through gait analysis is extremely important. Two high-profile studies performed over a decade ago (Noonan et al. 2003; Gorton et al. 2009) documented unacceptable levels of variability between different gait analysts (in different clinical services). The clinical gait analysis community has responded admirably to this challenge, and more recent studies (summarised in McGinley et al. 2009) report more acceptable levels of measurement variability. The quality of most of those measurements, however, is extremely dependent on the techniques employed by the staff of the gait analysis service, and constant vigilance is required to ensure that the quality of measurements made in routine clinical practice is of the same high level as that reported in this literature. Chapter 11 outlined steps that can be taken to ensure the quality of data that can be incorporated into the routine practice of data collection and analysis. This chapter describes additional exercises that should be implemented outside routine service provision to assure data quality.

Through any discussion of accuracy or repeatability, it is important to hold some idea of how much measurement variability is acceptable. This will depend on the context of how the data are being used. Clearly the smaller the effects that are assumed to be clinically significant, the lower the acceptable variability. In the context of conventional use of gait analysis data, McGinley et al. (2009) have suggested that total measurement variability of less than 2° is likely to be regarded as *acceptable* and will not need to be considered explicitly when interpreting data. Variability of between 2° and 5° is *reasonable* but will need to be considered in interpretation. Variability of over 5° is *concerning* and may be large enough to mislead interpretation.

Accuracy

The ultimate test of any measuring system is whether it is accurate or not. Unfortunately, this has an implicit requirement of having a better measurement system, a *criterion standard,* with which to compare it. Given the rigid segment biomechanical models that are used in gait analysis, it is clear that relevant criterion standards are measures of how the bones move during walking. Uniplanar or biplanar fluoroscopy can provide this but only under limited circumstances. The field of view of current systems is small, and so far measurements have been limited to the knee during treadmill walking (Fantozzi et al. 2003; Tsai et al. 2009; Akbarshahi et al. 2010). Concerns relating to radiation exposure place severe limitations on the amount of data from any individual, prevent the use on children and of scans of the pelvis (to avoid irradiating the genitalia). Current techniques require a computed tomography or magnetic resonance imaging (MRI) of the bones to register with the fluoroscopic image that increases the cost. The complexity of the bones of the foot makes such registration challenging. There are also considerable challenges in positioning motion capture cameras appropriately to see markers around the bulky equipment.

Open dynamic MRI has been used to detect meniscal movement during knee movement (Vedi et al. 1999) and low-dose biplanar digital radiography (Dubousset et al. 2005) to provide three-dimensional modelling of bones in a standing position. There is, however, little immediate prospect of either technology being developed sufficiently to image bone movements during walking. Ultrasound has also been used for measuring the hip joint centre (Hicks and Richards 2005; Peters et al. 2010; Sangeux et al. 2011), but its suitability for more general applications is not obvious.

Bone pins (Reinschmidt et al. 1997; Ramsey et al. 2003; Benoit et al. 2007; Nester et al. 2007; Rozumalski et al. 2008) and percutaneous trackers (Manal et al. 2003; Houck et al. 2004) have been used to validate biomechanical models of walking. They can certainly be used to ascertain whether technical markers move in relation to the underlying bone but have limited application to the more challenging issue of how the anatomical frames are defined. Indeed one bone pin study of knee movement (Benoit et al. 2006) shows knee adduction traces looking suspiciously like the artefact observed in gait analysis when the coronal plane of the femur has been identified incorrectly during anatomical calibration.

In summary, these techniques have considerable technical limitations, are expensive and are not widely available. They may be useful in developing and validating new modelling approaches, but it is unlikely that they will be developed to provide criterion standards by which the accuracy of clinical gait analysis can be judged in the foreseeable future.

Comparison of normative data

In the absence of criterion standards, perhaps the best technique available to assess the validity of data collected within a particular clinical gait analysis service is to compare the data collected from a cohort of people with no neuromusculoskeletal pathology to the data from similar cohorts collected in different centres. Figure 13.1 shows the mean and standard deviation of a cohort of children from one centre (Schwartz and Rozumalski 2008) plotted over standard deviation bands from another centre (Baker et al. 2009).

The good general agreement in both mean values and standard deviations suggests measurement practices are consistent. Where differences do exist, they can be related to known differences in detailed marker placement procedures.

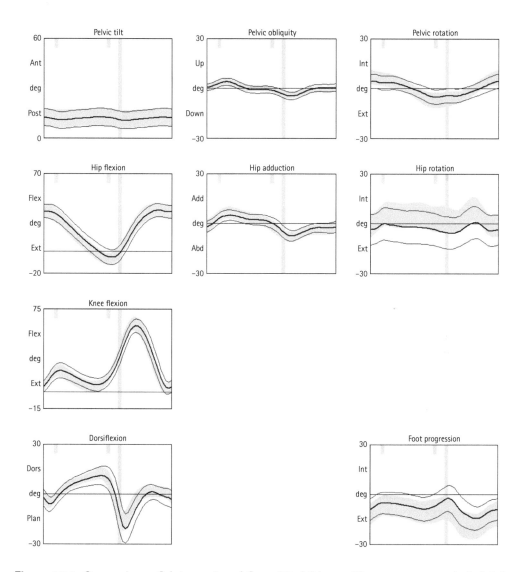

Figure 13.1 Comparison of data captured from 38 children with no neuromusculoskeletal pathology in one centre (Baker et al. 2009) and 166 similar limbs from another (Schwartz and Rozumalski 2008) showing excellent agreement for most traces; some discrepancies between dorsiflexion and foot progression are a consequence of minor differences in placement of the forefoot marker and an offset of about 5° in hip rotation arises from different techniques for calculating the thigh rotation offset.

Whilst clinical gait analysis was in the development phase, it was assumed that measurements would vary between different centres depending on the particular procedures they adopted. It was important to collect normative data to ensure that patient data were compared with reference data captured using exactly the same procedures. Now that the field has moved into a consolidation phase, and particularly now that a consensus is developing in how coordinate systems should be defined (see Chapters 3 and 4) this is no longer acceptable. Patients and referring clinicians are entitled to expect that wherever measurements are made they are compatible. The reason for collecting normative data in the modern world should be to compare with those collected at other centres to ensure that techniques are consistent. This should be tested at the level of individual analysts within centres as well as between centres.

Unfortunately national and international organisations have been slow to organise frameworks for such a process and such comparative studies are rare. In the absence of data collected specifically for this purpose, that downloadable as supplementary material to Schwartz and Rozumalski (2008) through *Gait and Posture* is the most authoritative source of such data for the conventional gait model. Cohorts do not need to be particularly big for comparisons to be useful. The standard error of the mean is the standard deviation divided by the square root of the sample size. Most clinically useful kinematic variables have standard deviations of less than 6°, and a cohort of just 10 people will specify the standard error of the mean to within 2° (=6°/$\sqrt{10}$). There has been very little work on whether gait kinematics or kinetics vary across the world for genetic or cultural reasons (or indeed as a consequence of age or sex). Clearly such comparisons are only valid if the gait patterns of the different cohorts can be regarded as similar, and more research is required to quantify the magnitude of any such differences. Consideration of the data presented in Figure 13.1, however, suggests strongly that the characteristics of the two cohorts are similar and that differences can be attributed mainly to measurement technique.

Measurement variability

Gait analysis data are particularly susceptible to measurement variability. Formal definitions of the anatomical landmarks which guide marker placement are improving (van Sint Jan 2007), but it is still difficult to palpate these through skin and other soft tissues and place markers precisely, which leads in turn to variability in kinematic and kinetic measurements. In order to avoid misinterpreting clinical data, it is essential to understand how much variability is associated with these measurements. Because this is fundamentally a consequence of the technique of individual analysts, it is essential that this quantified for individual analysts.

Comparing the mean traces for cohorts of people with no neuromusculoskeletal impairments only gives an indication of whether there are any systematic differences between how measurements are made in different centres. Comparing the standard deviations from such exercises gives some indication of measurement variability. Therefore in Figure 13.1 standard deviations are similar except for measures of hip rotation where they are 30% larger for one centre. This suggests higher measurement variability for this particular variable. Because there is considerable natural variability in the gait patterns of people with no neuromusculoskeletal impairments, however, this method cannot provide the direct measures of variability which are essential to guide clinical interpretation. Specific repeatability studies are essential, and there is no alternative to making repeat measurements on the same individual.

Variance components
The fundamental measure of variability is the *standard error of measurement* (SEM) (Stratford and Goldsmith 1997). There are a variety of ways of calculating this, but it is, essentially, an estimate of the standard deviation of a number of repeat measures on an individual person. Therefore 68% of measurements will lie within one SEM of the mean value (and consequently 32% will lie outside this). The main aim of a repeatability study is to obtain an estimate of the SEM. If that value is considered too high, however, further analysis is possible to identify where this is coming from and therefore to indicate how the SEM can be reduced.

The SEM can be considered to arise from various sources. In gait analysis, the main sources will be

(1) *within-analyst variability* (s_{WA}) arising because of random differences in marker placement whenever a particular analyst applies a marker set,
(2) *between-analyst variability* (s_{BA}) arising because of systematic differences between the way different analysts place markers,
(3) *between-trial variability* (s_{BT}) arising because the patient walks differently every time data are captured.[1]

The within-analyst variability can be calculated either as a specific value for each analyst or as an average across a number of different analysts.

Because of the way these quantities are calculated, it is actually the square of these terms that are added together. This quantity is called the *variance* (s^2), and hence the different sources of variability are referred to as *variance components*. These are related to the SEM by

$$\text{SEM} = \sqrt{s_{WA}^2 + s_{BA}^2 + s_{BT}^2}$$

---

[1] There may be some variability between the way people walk when they attend on different occasions over and above the between-trial variability. An unpublished study (McGinley and Baker) performed on young adults with no neuromusculoskeletal pathology suggested that this was very small ($\sim 1°$). In practice, it is virtually impossible to distinguish from within-analyst variability and so is generally considered a subcomponent of this.

Study design – principles

The basic principle of repeatability studies is quite simple. A number of analysts are required to make repeat measurements on a number of people. Such studies are performed to estimate the probable variability arising in routine clinical practice and should therefore be conducted under circumstances as similar to that practice as possible. This should involve the use of routine equipment, techniques and methods of data processing and modelling. A particular issue is the time between repeat assessments. Analysts are likely to retain some memory of marker placement if this is too short, and therefore estimates of the SEM will not reflect routine practice.

The main determinant of measurement variability in gait analysis is marker placement error. This is likely to be influenced by spasticity contracture, spasticity, bony deformity, cognitive impairment and behavioural problems, and ideal studies would therefore be conducted on patients typical of those encountered in clinical practice. Such studies are quite difficult to organise, and the extent to which such factors affect measurement is unknown. Studies on people with no neuromusculoskeletal pathology are more practical and are certainly better than no studies at all. The most important feature is probably the amount of subcutaneous soft tissue, and the temptation to select leaner people for repeatability studies should be resisted. It is also possible that fixed absolute errors in marker placement will have a larger effect on joint angles in smaller individuals, and therefore repeatability studies for use in paediatric gait analysis should probably be conducted with children.

The confidence with which the SEM can be estimated is determined by the total number of repeat measurements made. Most study designs result in a large number of repeat measurements, and therefore the SEM can be estimated with some confidence. The within- and between-assessor variance components, however, depend principally on the number of people and sessions. These are generally limited by practical considerations. A minimum of three sessions and three people is probably required for any confidence in the variance components estimates. Smaller studies can still provide useful information, but results should not be overinterpreted. If resources are available, the focus should be on increasing the number of people. Although it is relatively easy to collect a large number of trials at each session, this adds little to increase confidence in results.

Despite explicit steps to avoid it, repeatability studies are almost always conducted under somewhat idealised conditions, and staff will also probably be especially vigilant while making assessments. Estimates of variability obtained from studies will therefore almost always underestimate the variability in routine clinical practice, and this should be remembered when applying results to clinical interpretation.

Study design – practice

Most clinical gait analysis services employ a small number of analysts, and it is generally practical to have each analyst make measurements on all individuals at the same number of sessions (Figure 13.2). For three analysts making measurements at three sessions on each of three people requires 27 measurement sessions. This sounds formidable but given that the focus on each session is purely on placing markers this can be streamlined much more than analyses conducted for clinical purposes. Figure 13.3 illustrates how three analysts could each measure three people in a single session. This could be repeated at two other sessions each a week apart. Such regimes can be quite demanding on the person being analysed and may not be suitable for young children. They also require a second marker set, which is a useful investment for such exercises. Obviously the exact way that such exercises are planned will depend on local circumstances.

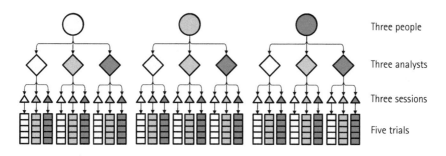

Figure 13.2 Experimental design for a repeatability study (Figure from Schwartz et al. 2004 with permission).

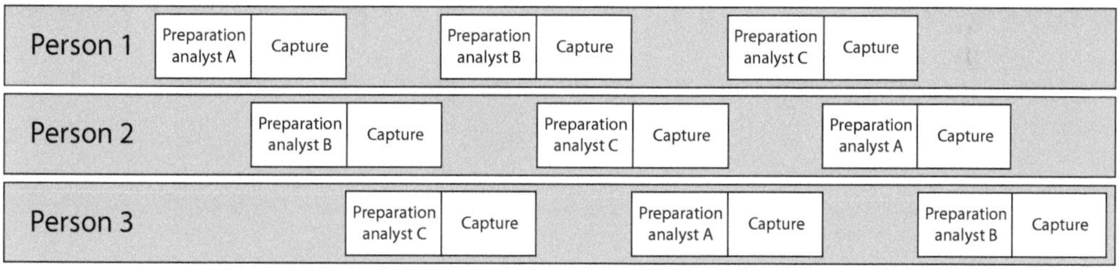

Person 1	Preparation analyst A	Capture		Preparation analyst B	Capture		Preparation analyst C	Capture
Person 2			Preparation analyst B	Capture		Preparation analyst C	Capture	Preparation analyst A	Capture
Person 3					Preparation analyst C	Capture		Preparation analyst A	Capture	Preparation analyst B	Capture

Figure 13.3 Planning so that three analysts can measure three people in one session making good use of time and facilities.

Repeatability studies are time-consuming, but they are perhaps the best currently available method for quantifying and understanding measurement error within individual services. Given that high-quality measurements are the essential prerequisite for any subsequent interpretation of data, time invested in these exercises is well spent. An appropriate balance is probably to conduct such studies across all analysts once each year (although taking so much time might be difficult to justify for part-time staff). Smaller less formal tests can be extremely informative and might be conducted more frequently. Thus between-analyst consistency could be based on comparing data from each analyst capturing data on one individual on one occasion. It is also important to involve new staff in similar studies to ensure that their performance is consistent with other staff. A full study need not be conducted across all staff, but several informal bilateral comparisons between the new analyst and different established analysts can be informative. Even if there is only one analyst employed in a given service, it is useful to perform studies to give confidence that he or she is making consistent measurements.

Repeatability studies are essentially a means of quantifying how well analysts place markers. They can therefore be a source of some apprehension for those analysts. Whilst an open discussion of results within the team is almost certainly the most effective way to use such studies to improve measurements, some thought should be given as to how results will first be presented back to analysts. This is obviously a particular issue if results suggest that some analysts are more variable in their technique than others. Presenting individual analysts with their own data and the team with anonymised data is one way of handling this.

Presenting the results of repeatability studies

Perhaps the most useful form of presenting the results of repeatability studies in gait analysis are plots of variability from different sources across the gait cycle (see Figure 13.4) (Schwartz et al. 2004). Schwartz et al. used a slightly different approach to that outlined above in that they calculated the cumulative variance (i.e. inter-therapist variability includes that for session and trial), and in this context the inter-therapist variability equates to the SEM. The data therefore give a clear indication of the SEM and how different sources of variability contribute to this.

Gait reliability profiles

Measurement variability in gait kinematics does not vary much across the gait cycle (Schwartz et al. 2004), and therefore values averaged across the gait cycle are generally

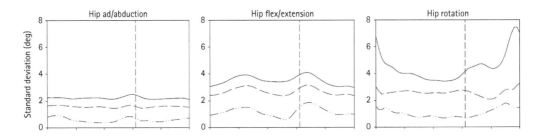

Figure 13.4 Variance components plotted across the gait cycle (Figure from Schwartz et al. 2004 with permission). It should be noted that this uses a slightly different approach to this variance analysis in that the inter-session variance is not separated from the inter-therapist variance but is included within it (and similarly for the inter-trial and inter-session variances).

all that are required. Standard errors of measurement for the clinically important joint angles can be plotted as a bar chart, which has been referred to as a *gait reliability profile* (GRP, see McGinley et al. 2006). Additional information regarding variance components have been superimposed upon this. The dark grey area is the procedural variability that arises from how analysts place markers ($= \sqrt{s_{WA}^2 + s_{BA}^2}$). The lighter grey area on top of this represents the additional variability that arises from inter-trial variability. The horizontal bars represent the between (black) and within (white) analyst variability. For the data depicted here, the between-analyst variance is high for most angles, suggesting that improvements are most likely to come from working on consistency between analysts. The one exception to this is hip adduction in which within-analyst variability is higher, suggesting that the limiting factor here is how repeatably individual analysts place markers but that within this there is little inconsistency between analysts. It is possible to generate similar graphs for individual analysts, but these will not have between- or within-analyst data (see Figure 13.5).

Overplotting data
Whilst the GRP summarises where variability is occurring (which joint angles and whether it is arising between or within analysts), it gives little specific information as to how variability arises. If there is large between-analyst variability within a centre, for example, it is useful to know whether this arises because all analysts are using a slightly different technique or most are consistent with one showing marked differences. Perhaps the easiest way to examine this is to plot gait data from the different sources in different colours. Therefore in Figure 13.6 data from three analysts have been plotted. It can be

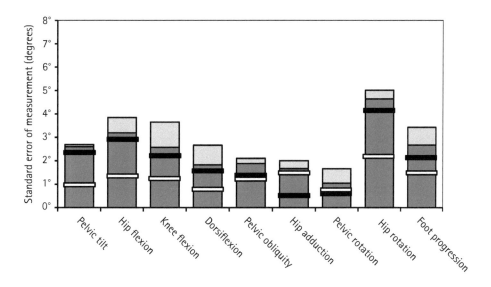

Figure 13.5 Gait reliability profile (see the text for explanation).

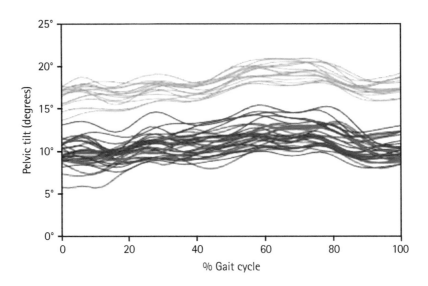

Figure 13.6 Pelvic tilt data from one person measured by three analysts at each of two sessions. Data from each analyst have been plotted in a different colour regardless of session.

seen that the red and blue analysts show consistent practice while the green analyst has been placing markers in a way that results in approximately 10° more pelvic tilt being recorded. Training is clearly required to improve consistency between analysts. The data here are colour coded with respect to analyst, but a greater range of colours can be used to code for session and/or patient as well.

Repeatability studies in the literature
Several formal studies have quantified measurement repeatability in gait analysis. These have been reviewed by (McGinley et al. 2009) and the results are presented in Figure 13.7. The data show that the variability differs from joint to joint and across planes. Most joints show variability of 4° or less, with the exception of hip rotation. Whilst six of the studies show hip rotation variability of greater than 6°, five show variability of around 4° or less, suggesting some difference in variability at different centres. Using the criteria established above suggests that most measurements fall in the 'reasonable' category (between 2° and 5°) and therefore require to be considered when interpreting data. Particular care is required in relation to hip rotation to maintain variability within these limits, and there is evidence of 'concerning' levels of variability from some studies. It is worth noting that these studies are reporting less measurement variability than in comparable studies of physical examination measurements (McDowell et al. 2000; Fosang et al. 2003). If clinicians have confidence in physical exam measurements as a basis for clinical decision-making, then they should have even more confidence in clinical gait analysis.

Presenting the results of repeatability studies as the SEM and subdividing this into different variance components results in measurements that are reported in the same units as the measurements themselves (see Figure 13.7). The relevance to clinical interpretation is generally immediately obvious. Clearly the greater the difference between two gait traces

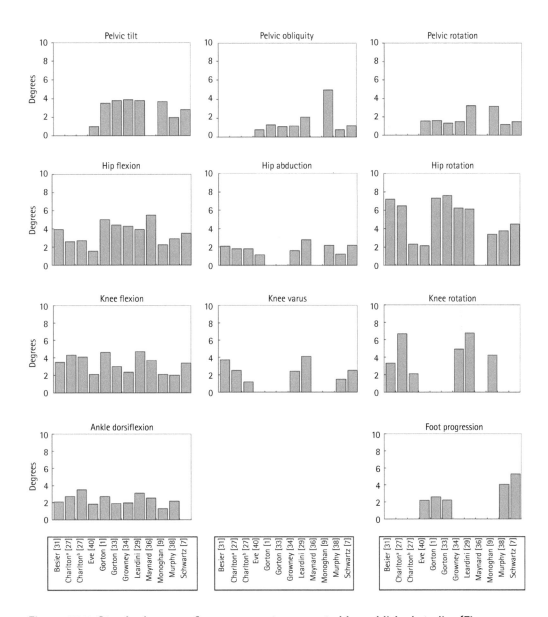

Figure 13.7 Standard errors of measurement as reported by published studies (Figure from McGinley et al. 2009 with permission).

(either that from a patient and the mean of the normative database, or two traces from the same person at different times) compared to the SEM then the more confidence we have that this is real and not just a consequence of measurement variability. Reporting the results of repeatability studies in this way has considerable advantages over other measures that are prevalent in the literature but should generally be avoided (see Appendix 2).

References

Akbarshahi M, Schache AG, Fernandez JW, Baker R, Banks S, Pandy MG. Non-invasive assessment of soft-tissue artifact and its effect on knee joint kinematics during functional activity. *J Biomech*, 2010, 43:1292–1301. DOI: 10.1016/j.jbiomech.2010.01.002

Baker R, McGinley JL, Schwartz MH et al. The gait profile score and movement analysis profile. *Gait Posture*, 2009, 30:265–269. DOI: 10.1016/j.gaitpost.2009.05.020

Benoit DL, Ramsey DK, Lamontagne M, Xu L, Wretenberg P, Renström P. Effect of skin movement artifact on knee kinematics during gait and cutting motions measured in vivo. *Gait Posture*, 2006, 24:152–164.

Benoit DL, Ramsey DK, Lamontagne M, Xu L, Wretenberg P, Renström P. In vivo knee kinematics during gait reveals new rotation profiles and smaller translations. *Clin Orthop Relat Res*, 2007, 454:81–88.

Dubousset J, Charpak G, Dorion I et al. A new 2D and 3D imaging approach to musculoskeletal physiology and pathology with low-dose radiation and the standing position: the EOS system. *Bull Acad Natl Med*, 2005, 189:287–297; discussion 297–300.

Fantozzi S, Benedetti MG, Leardini A et al. Fluoroscopic and gait analysis of the functional performance in stair ascent of two total knee replacement designs. *Gait Posture*, 2003, 17:225–234.

Fosang AL, Galea MP, McCoy AT, Reddihough DS, Story I. Measures of muscle and joint performance in the lower limb of children with cerebral palsy. *Dev Med Child Neurol*, 2003, 45:664–670.

Gorton GE, 3rd, Hebert DA, Gannotti ME. Assessment of the kinematic variability among 12 motion analysis laboratories. *Gait Posture*, 2009, 29:398–402. DOI: 10.1016/j.gaitpost.2008.10.060

Hicks JL, Richards JG. Clinical applicability of using spherical fitting to find hip joint centers. *Gait Posture*, 2005, 22:138–145. DOI: 10.1016/j.gaitpost.2004.08.004

Houck J, Yack HJ, Cuddeford T. Validity and comparisons of tibiofemoral orientations and displacement using a femoral tracking device during early to mid stance of walking. *Gait Posture*, 2004, 19:76–84. DOI: 10.1016/S0966-6362(03)00033-X

Manal K, McClay Davis I, Galinat B, Stanhope S. The accuracy of estimating proximal tibial translation during natural cadence walking: bone vs. skin mounted targets. *Clin Biomech (Bristol, Avon)*, 2003, 18:126–131.

McDowell BC, Hewitt V, Nurse A, Weston T, Baker RJ. The variability of goniometric measurements in ambulatory children with spastic cerebral palsy. *Gait Posture*, 2000, 12:114–121. DOI: 10.1016/S0966-6362(00)00068-0

McGinley J, Baker R, Wolfe R. Quantification of kinematic measurement variability in gait analysis. *Gait Posture*, 2006, 24:S55–56.

McGinley JL, Baker R, Wolfe R, Morris ME. The reliability of three–dimensional kinematic gait measurements: a systematic review. *Gait Posture*, 2009, 29:360–369. DOI: 10.1016/j.gaitpost.2008.09.003

Nester C, Jones RK, Liu A et al. Foot kinematics during walking measured using bone and surface mounted markers. *J Biomech*, 2007, 40:3412–3423. DOI: 10.1016/j.jbiomech.2007.05.019

Noonan K, Halliday S, Browne R, O'Brien S, Kayes K, Feinberg J. Inter-observer variability of gait analysis in patients with cerebral palsy. *J Pediatr Orthop*, 2003, 23:279–287.

Peters A, Baker R, Sangeux M. Validation of 3-D freehand ultrasound for the determination of the hip joint centre. *Gait Posture*, 2010, 31:530–532. DOI: 10.1016/j.gaitpost.2010.01.014

Ramsey DK, Wretenberg PF, Benoit DL, Lamontagne M, Németh G. Methodological concerns using intra-cortical pins to measure tibiofemoral kinematics. *Knee Surg, Sport Tr, A*, 2003, 11:344–349.

Reinschmidt C, van Den Bogert AJ, Murphy N, Lundberg A, Nigg BM. Tibiocalcaneal motion during running, measured with external and bone markers. *Clin Biomech (Bristol, Avon)*, 1997, 12:8–16. DOI: 10.1016/S0268-0033(96)00046-0

Rozumalski A, Schwartz MH, Wervy R, Swanson A, Dykes DC, Novacheck T. The in vivo three-dimensional motion of the human lumbar spine during gait. *Gait Posture*, 2008, 28:378–384. DOI: 10.1016/j.gaitpost.2008.05.005

Sangeux M, Peters A, Baker R Hip joint centre localization: evaluation on normal subjects in the context of gait analysis. *Gait Posture*, 2011, 34:324–328. DOI: 10.1016/j.gaitpost.2011.05.019

Schwartz MH, Rozumalski A The gait deviation index: a new comprehensive index of gait pathology. *Gait Posture*, 2008, 28:351–357. DOI: 10.1016/j.gaitpost.2008.05.001

Schwartz MH, Trost JP, Wervey RA Measurement and management of errors in quantitative gait data *Gait Posture*, 2004, 20:196–203. DOI: 10.1016/j.gaitpost.2003.09.011

Stratford PW, Goldsmith CH. Use of the standard error as a reliability index of interest: an applied example using elbow flexor strength data *Phys Ther*, 1997, 77:745–750.

Tsai T-Y, Lu T-W, Kuo M-Y, Hsu H-C. Quantification of three-dimensional movement of skin markers realtive to the underlying bones during functional activities. *Biomed Eng Appl, Basis Commun*, 2009, 21:223–232. DOI: 10.4015/S1016237209001283

van Sint Jan S. *Color Atlas of Skeletal Landmark Definitions: Guidelines for Reproducible Manual and Virtual Palpations.* London: Churchill Livingstone, 2007.

Vedi V, Williams A, Tennant SJ, Spouse E, Hunt DM, Gedroyc WM. Meniscal movement. An in-vivo study using dynamic MRI. *J Bone Joint Surg Br*, 1999, 81:37–41.

Chapter 14

How to set up a clinical gait analysis service

Clinical governance

Clinical governance is a system through which [healthcare] organisations are account-able for continuously improving the quality of their services and safeguarding high standards of care by creating an environment in which excellence in clinical care will flourish.

(Scally and Donaldson 1998)

Like all other clinical services, modern clinical gait analysis needs to operate within a rigorous framework of clinical governance. At a bare minimum, this needs to ensure that services are delivered safely, legally and ethically, but, as reflected in the definition above, there is an increasing emphasis on creating an environment in which excellence can flourish rather than one in which minimum standards are simply adhered to. In the context of clinical gait analysis, this framework needs to ensure that measurements are accurate and representative of the individual patient and that any interpretation of the data is transparent, evidence based and within the competence of those performing the interpretation. Services need to be operated with regard to the safety, comfort and dignity of the patient and, in the case of children, of their families.

There is an increasing understanding that all healthcare providers, regardless of whether they operate from within a conventional healthcare institution or not, need to function within such a framework. In many countries, this is now embedded within legislation. In England, for example, it is now a legal requirement for all providers of healthcare services to register with the Care Quality Commission (CQC) and in doing so need to provide evidence of the framework of clinical governance that they have in place.

Staffing

Clinical gait analysis services require a range of skills:

Director: Someone needs to give overall direction to the service. This is a high-level function and the director will generally also act as the primary advocate for the service within the host organisation. This role is most often filled by a senior surgeon or other clinician.

Manager: Even a fairly small gait analysis service will require someone to take care of day-to-day management. This is generally too detailed and time consuming to be suitable for the director and most services appoint a separate manager. This will be a senior appointment of someone who could come from a range of professional backgrounds. If the person is new to management, they may require specific training in management techniques.

Gait analyst: The gait analyst takes responsibility for the gait analysis. That person should have a thorough knowledge of the measurements made, covering all of the issues covered in this book. The person also needs to be experienced in working with patients and have qualifications and registration with an appropriate professional body to reflect this. In most countries, a physiotherapist or kinesiologist fills this role.

Biomechanist: Gait analysis services often find it useful to employ a biomechanist to take responsibility for the measurement equipment and to provide expert input to interpretation. Few countries have formal training schemes to equip staff for such a role, and as a consequence they can come from a variety of backgrounds. (The United Kingdom is an exception with formal training of clinical engineers leading to state registration.)

Technician: Clinical gait analysis generally requires a second person to be present during the conduct of assessments. Such a person can be extremely useful for supporting the gait analyst in performing a physical examination and is essential to support data capture. There is generally also a requirement for significant postcapture data processing prior to interpretation. (This is partly a consequence of the complexity of current data capture and analysis software. In the future, it is possible that developments in such software could reduce the need for such support.)

Clinician: If a service is providing clinical recommendations as well as a biomechanical analysis, then it is essential to have appropriately trained staff who are qualified to do so. Therefore if surgical recommendations are being made, then a surgeon should be involved or if physiotherapy is being recommended then a physiotherapist should be involved. (It is surprisingly common to find services who make such recommendations without having appropriately qualified staff involved.)

Clerical officer: Whilst patient throughput in gait analysis is typically quite low, the appointment procedure can often be complex. Patients generally have a range of disabilities and appointments may need co-ordinating with other departments. Because each appointment lasts for several hours, failure to attend is a considerable waste of staff and laboratory time and it makes sense to do everything possible to facilitate attendance. This person can also handle billing, staff rosters, filing, typing, mailing, etc.

How any particular service achieves this skill mix within its staff varies greatly from place to place (see Figures 14.1 and 14.2). Gait analysis is too small a profession to justify specific undergraduate training, and professionals involved in gait analysis tend to come from a range of backgrounds and have a varying mix of individual experience and skills. Smaller services almost always appoint staff to fulfil more than one of the above roles. It is common to find a manager who doubles as a gait analyst or biomechanist or a biomechanist who doubles as a technician. Where appropriate registration is possible, more consideration should be given to training people with a biomechanics background to take on the full gait analyst role outlined above. In smaller services, the clerical officer's role might be carried out by one of the other staff.

Clinical governance requires clear lines of accountability which are most conveniently summarised in an organisational chart. It also requires clear allocation of responsibilities which are specified in position descriptions for each member of staff. It is fairly common to have staff who share part-time responsibilities in the gait analysis service with other responsibilities elsewhere in the host organisation. If this is the case, it can be extremely useful to have a specific position descriptions for the different roles. A further issue is that of professional accountability. Line management structures can involve staff from one professional group being managed by staff from a different group. It can be useful to specifically designate a parallel line manager to manage any professional issues that might arise.

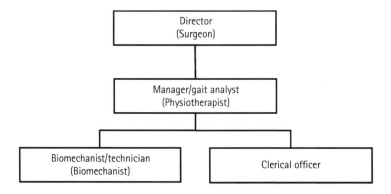

Figure 14.1 Organisation chart for a small service.

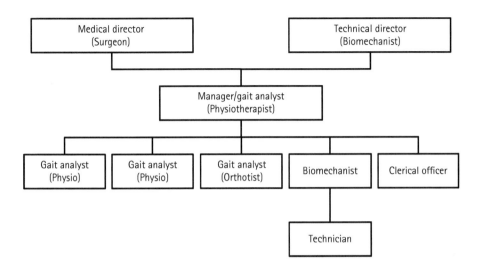

Figure 14.2 Organisation chart for a larger service.

Maintaining the skill mix within a gait analysis service can be a major challenge. Organisational structures often evolve to optimise the competencies of individual members of staff. This can create problems when staff leave as finding an individual to exactly replicate the role of the previous staff member can be extremely difficult. Some larger gait analysis services have developed to a stage where a fixed organisational structure is viable on an ongoing basis, but many smaller services need to review their structure whenever a key member of staff is replaced to ensure optimum use of staff talents.

Ensuring career progression options for staff can be a particular challenge. It is quite common to appoint relatively senior staff to specialist positions but then have no options to recognise progress within the post. This can be exacerbated by lack of movement higher up the organisational structure. Specialist roles can often appear exciting and challenging when staff are first appointed and learning the role. Once this period is over, however, the roles may become more routine, and this may lead to frustration for staff who have enjoyed the challenge and stimulation of learning their new roles. Staff specialising in gait analysis might become de-skilled for their original role and may find difficulty moving to other roles even if they want to.

Recruiting appropriate staff is the most important determinant of the quality of a gait analysis service. The service manager is an extremely important role. There are particular difficulties here when creating a new service. In an ideal world, the manager would be appointed early in the process and have significant involvement in designing facilities and deciding on equipment purchases. Lead times, particularly on building projects, however, are such that the cost of such early recruitment can generally not be justified. Particular care must therefore be taken by project drivers to ensure that appropriate advice is obtained to ensure that major decisions are well founded and that all plans are well matched to project aims.

Procedures

Level of service

There are two broad levels of service delivery within gait analysis services. In the first, a comprehensive assessment is conducted leading to treatment recommendations. Such recommendations generally require considerably more information than is required for the gait analysis itself. The psychosocial background of the patient (and carers) may need to be assessed before recommending some complex interventions, for example. Obviously the clinical interview and examination will need to be extended to capture such information.

In the second, the analysis is restricted to a purely biomechanical analysis of the patient without explicit treatment recommendations. This can be achieved with a much more focused biomechanical assessment. Services need to decide which of these two they are offering and plan assessments accordingly. If treatment recommendations are being made, then it is essential that only staff trained and qualified to make such recommendations do so. It is also worth reflecting whether this is the best approach for the patient. A child's long-standing community physiotherapist might be better placed to comment on the psychosocial background than a gait analysis service physiotherapist at the end of a short interview. It should also be remembered that treatment recommendations depend not only on the assessment of the patient but also on the experience, skills and preferences of the clinician and the facilities available to him or her.

Referrals

Gait analysis is an expensive and time-consuming process, and systems are required to ensure that only patients who are likely to benefit are assessed. At the very least, there should be clear guidance readily available for potential referring clinicians to understand the strengths and limitations of gait analysis. A safer process is for patients to be referred to a preliminary consultation with a clinician who is part of the gait analysis team to assess whether they are likely to benefit from a full analysis.

Modern systems can cope with even the smallest children; so the lower age limit is generally determined by the child's ability to co-operate with the assessment process. A lower age limit of five will generally ensure this, although some services will accept referrals of younger children. The patient must also be able to walk the length of the walkway several times.

It is useful if the referrer states specifically why he is referring a patient and what questions he would like the analysis to answer. It is extremely difficult, however, to ensure that referrers are so specific and procedures should not be dependent upon this.

Appointments

Many patients will not have heard of gait analysis before their referral, and sending a short explanatory leaflet with the appointment letter can be most useful. Patients should be forewarned about the extent to which they will be required to undress and whether any particular clothing is required. Shorts (not long or baggy) and a T-shirt are recommended. Some centres suggest swim suits, but one-piece female swim suits prevent markers being attached to the skin over the pelvic landmarks. It is worth restating the referral criteria in case an inappropriate referral has been made. Gait analysis takes much longer than many other hospital appointments, and the expected duration of the appointment should also be clearly stated.

Given the resources in terms of personnel and laboratory time that can be wasted by failure to attend, it is sensible to actively consult patients to agree an appointment time in advance of sending a confirmatory letter.

Data capture
Specific protocols for data capture will be determined by the equipment used and will not be described in detail. One particular issue though is what combination of shoes and orthoses and/or walking aids should be used. Capturing data under multiple conditions can be extremely time consuming. Choice of conditions will depend on the reasons for the referral, but the focus of the analysis is generally to establish the inherent capability of the patient, and this suggests walking with minimal supports (bare feet and the minimum walking aids to achieve a reasonable gait pattern). It may also be useful to assess how the patient walks in everyday situations (shoes, orthoses and normal walking aids).

Interpretation and reporting
The level of reporting depends on the level of service being offered (see Section 4.1) and involves appropriate staff. Some centres actually supply two reports, the first being a biomechanical interpretation provided by the gait analyst and the second being treatment recommendations provided by a senior clinician (who may, occasionally, also have been the gait analyst). A biomechanical interpretation of data can be conducted by a staff with a good understanding of the relevant biomechanical issues. Treatment recommendations, however, should only be made by clinicians appropriately qualified to do so. There is a subjective element to almost all biomechanical interpretation, and reporting should be sufficiently transparent to allow the referring clinician to understand how the conclusions have been arrived at. It is good practice to include copies of the data with the report.

In many centres, a technician processes and formats data prior to interpretation, and a gait analyst then performs a preliminary interpretation which is then discussed either with a team or with a senior clinician. It is extremely useful to have a specialist biomechanist available to assist with the biomechanical analysis and interpretation.

Economics

Costs
There are a variety of different costs associated with gait analysis. The most significant is staff time. High costs are a result of a combination of high salaries for staff with specific clinical skills and the considerable workload associated with each assessment.

Equipment costs can also be high. In past years, this has been exacerbated by a perceived need to upgrade hardware fairly regularly, with some centres upgrading as often as every 3 years. Until recently, upgrades have conferred substantial improvements in data quality, and such upgrades have seemed sensible. System performance is now such that it is difficult to see how clinical measurement will be improved by future hardware development, and there may be less need for regular upgrades. Many hospitals are developing more sophisticated models for calculating facilities costs. A particular issue for gait analysis is that some are starting to levy a charge based on the floor area of any facility. Gait analysis has a high ratio of floor area to throughput and can be badly affected by such a system.

Income

Clinical gait analysis services are funded in a variety of different ways. Some are simply funded from the hospital's operating budget. Others have block funding from outside the hospital simply to deliver a clinical gait analysis service or to deliver it to a target number of patients. Such funding generally comes from a national or local government source. Probably the most common funding model is for a charge to be raised for each patient assessed. Such charges can be paid by the individual, a health insurance organisation, a health commissioner or local or national government. In some countries, a national price has been set for gait analysis through some system or other. In most, however, gait analysis services are free to negotiate a price with the purchasers of gait analysis.

Balancing the books

Gait analysis is an expensive business. In many countries, the cost of a gait analysis can be up to three times that of a magnetic resonance imaging scan. There is no doubt that this price is a barrier to use. It is difficult to justify using gait analysis to assess patients for less expensive treatment options. It is considerably cheaper, for example, to inject a child with cerebral palsy with botulinum toxin to see if it actually works than it is to refer them for a gait assessment to predict whether the toxin is likely to work. There is almost certainly huge potential for gait analysis to contribute to the management of stroke patients, but few resources are allocated to each patient for gait rehabilitation, and gait analysis will not be adopted unless assessment costs drop to be more in-line with rehabilitation costs.

Costs almost certainly can be reduced. The most obvious way is to increase throughput. Equipment and facilities charges are significant fixed costs that are shared by the number of patients being seen each year. The more patients, the lower the cost for each individual. Throughput can be reduced by using smarter working practices and in particularly by making appointments to ensure that laboratory facilities are used throughout the day. It is the laboratory itself that is most expensive, and preparing one patient in an assessment room while another is being assessed in the laboratory can increase throughput considerably.

Such steps, however, assume that there is a supply of referrals to fill laboratory time. Many laboratories are still used primarily for assessing children with cerebral palsy for complex surgery. The aim of such surgery is that it is only carried out once per child, and the prevalence of cerebral palsy is such that there are between 25 and 30 children born with the condition per million population per year. It is clear that clinical gait analysis services will have to cover a substantial population to fill available laboratory time with such assessments. Diversifying to supply services to different conditions is also clearly an option.

Staff time is the other large cost. Historically gait analysis services have employed relatively senior staff as gait analysis has been seen as a developmental activity which requires this. As procedures become more routine and standardised, it can be argued that it there is less need to employ such senior (and expensive) staff. Salary differentials, however, are relatively modest, and this is unlikely to lead to substantial savings.

The other factor is how much staff time is devoted to each patient. Most clinical gait analysis services will benefit from a critical analysis of how much time staff they spend with each patient and how many staff are in attendance at any one time. The time spent on interpretation and reporting of assessments varies substantially from centre to centre and in many could almost certainly be reduced if more focused and systematic approaches are adopted. It may also often be useful to review the time spent by staff on general tasks, which can result effectively in a substantial overhead for any service. Multi-person interdisciplinary interpretation and reporting sessions can be important drivers of high-quality outputs, but this needs to be balanced against the exceptional cost in terms of staff time. Ten people in a room for half a day costs as much as one person for a week (and such sessions generally include highly paid senior clinicians).

Many services augment patient-related income with income from other sources. The most obvious is research funding, given that the measurement equipment is extremely useful for outcome measurement. The demands of clinical research and clinical service delivery, however, can be quite different, and the best services remain highly aware of this when managing both in parallel. It is also reasonably common to find gait analysis services dependent on some source of philanthropic funds. This will typically be to fund new equipment or equipment upgrades.

Reference

Scally G, Donaldson L Clinical governance and the drive for quality improvement in the new NHS in England. *Br Med J*, 1998, 317:61–65. DOI: 10.1136/bmj.317.7150.61

Chapter 15
How to set up and maintain a gait analysis laboratory

General facilities and equipment

Gait analysis requires a reasonable space for making measurements. A walkway of 10m (with an additional 1m at each end for turning) should be regarded as a minimum length. Much better results will be obtained if the cameras are placed at a reasonable distance from the measuring volume and 8m should be regarded as the minimum width. It is worth noting that as hospital finances get more sophisticated, increasing numbers are including floor space in their model for costing facilities. Whilst more space might appear an advantage, it can result in substantial overheads being charged to the service.

Given the value of floor space within most hospitals, and the fact that many gait analysis services do not have sufficient throughput to require full-time use of the laboratory, it is tempting to consider dual use of the facilities. This is possible with planning. Solutions that require equipment, particularly cameras, to be stored somewhere between sessions should be avoided. Cameras fixed to walls or the ceiling can generally be positioned such that they can be left in place regardless of the use that is being made of the room. Force plates are quite resilient to routine activity particularly if covered by a mat. They need to be mounted below the floor level, which may require the floor level to be built up or a pit to be dug. There is a tendency for increasing numbers of force plates, and if a pit is required it should be big enough to allow for expansion. Although force plates require little maintenance, it should be possible to access them without having to damage the floor. A raised floor or false ceiling can be extremely useful for concealing cabling. A conduit will certainly be required for cabling from computer to the force plates. This should be wide enough to allow bulky connectors to be passed through as well as the cables.

Ensuring dignity and confidentiality for the patient is particularly important, and facilities should be arranged to allow patients to undress and dress in privacy and for any clinical interview or examination to be conducted confidentially. Having a separate area (or preferably room) for patient preparation and examination can be extremely useful (see Figure 15.1). In busier laboratories, use of a separate room offers the potential for one patient to be being prepared for gait analysis at the same time as another is actually having their assessment (having two preparation rooms adjoin the laboratory is even better). The service should have the sole use of facilities at the time of patient assessments regardless of what those facilities might be used for at other times. Having toilets that can be accessed by people with disabilities close to the laboratory can be extremely useful. A wash hand basin is essential in any clinical area where patients are being examined and a sharps bin may also be required particularly if fine wire EMG is practiced.

Consideration should be given to where patients and their carers are expected to wait prior to and during the appointment. Clearly some young children may need distraction whilst waiting. Many parents can be extremely supportive to clinical staff in encouraging

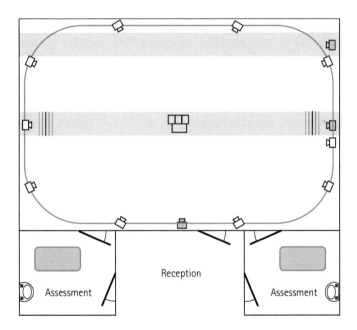

Figure 15.1 Ideal laboratory layout for a clinical service. One central walkway for motion capture using 10 cameras (white) mounted on ceiling rail around perimeter of room. Another walkway for video capture running along one wall to minimise parallax from sagittal plane camera. Three video cameras (in grey) wall mounted at about hip height. Force plates are located centrally and starting lines are placed symmetrically with regard to these. Separate assessment areas with independent access to both reception and that laboratory allow possibility to prepare one patient whilst conducting an analysis on the other. There should be a plinth and wash hand basin in both assessment rooms. A workstation and some seating for families can be placed in the corners of the laboratory.

their child to cooperate with procedures but this is not always the case. It is common for families to bring uninvolved siblings along to appointments and they need to be catered for. Toys which are too attractive however may distract the child being assessed. A sensible compromise is to have toys available but kept with containers unless required.

Walkways

Having a clearly defined walkway down the centre of the laboratory can be most useful. Defining this by using a floor covering different to the rest of the room is common. It can also be useful to have several different coloured parallel lines (around 10cm apart) marking the start of the walkway. This allows the patient to be started off at slightly different distances from the force plates to increase the chances of clean force plate strikes. Having these at both ends of the walkway at the same distances from the force plate should facilitate kinetic data collection when walking in both directions. The floor covering should have some compliance for comfort, given that many assessments require patients to walk in bare feet. It also needs to be easily cleanable. Matt surfaces can be useful to cut down reflections from the light sources of opposing cameras. Colour should be chosen to give good contrast with the skin if video is to be captured.

Many centres capture video synchronously with gait data, and clearly this requires the use of just one common walkway. Parallax on the video recording, however, is minimised by having the camera as far as possible from the patient, and the best quality video will therefore be obtained by having a second walkway along one side of the room. Whatever walkway is used, the background of the video should be as clean as possible. As with walkways, colour should be chosen to give good contrast with skin. Some markings on the walkway can be useful to allow step and stride length to be judged from video but should not be too obtrusive. Decorating the room to present a comfortable and welcoming environment is desirable, particularly in paediatric facilities. Understanding which areas will provide backdrop for video cameras will allow a variety of decorations on other wall areas. There are some fantastic examples of imaginative artwork adorning the walls of gait analysis facilities across the world.

Mounting cameras

Clinical gait analysis generally requires a fixed layout of cameras, which might only be modified occasionally (e.g. if extra cameras are purchased). Unless there is a specific requirement for flexibility, tripods are best avoided and cameras should be mounted on brackets attached to the walls or ceilings. Having a mounting rail running around the room close to the ceiling on which cameras can be mounted is probably the optimum set-up allowing for rigid mounting of cameras but some flexibility to adjust camera positions if the need arises.

Force plates

Manufacturers generally recommend that force plates are mounted on substantial foundations to reduce susceptibility to vibrations. This is most easily achieved in a ground floor facility. Installing force plates on other floors is possible but may impose specific structural requirements to support the concrete slab on which force plates need to be mounted. Some modern force plates are designed to be transportable and have less stringent requirements for mounting. Manufacturer's instructions should always be followed.

Force plates should be recessed into the floor wherever possible (even those that are designed to be transportable). Modern force plates are reasonably inexpensive given the other costs of establishing a gait analysis service and purchasing several can be extremely useful. Force plate layout is dependent on the characteristics of the patients being assessed. The aim is to maximise the chances of obtaining clean force plate strikes in which one foot is placed entirely within the surface of the plate and the other foot (or any walking aids) do not make contact with it at all. Most patients will put one foot a reasonable distance in front of the other and a single line of plates is probably the best arrangement. Some manufacturers allow signals from two plates to be added if the foot spans both (and the other foot or aids do not make contact with either). In this case, placing several plates in line with their edges abutting is most appropriate. The small number of patients who have very short step length often have a wide base of support and having one plate to the side of another can be extremely useful to obtain data (see Figure 15.2). It is virtually impossible to obtain valid force data from patients with short step length and narrow step width. When designing the layout, it should be remembered that patients generally have reduced stride length and that this will be a particular factor for children (children are also lighter and some manufacturers supply plates specifically designed for this).

Other equipment
Other equipment should be stored neatly and be readily accessible. Trolleys that can be wheeled into a position under a bench are ideal. Some centres like to make a feature of a workstation on which computers can be placed and behind which the technician can be seated. Others see this as unnecessarily intimidating, particularly if children and being assessed, and prefer a less formal arrangement. A standing frame can be exceedingly useful to support patients while they are having markers placed or performing functional calibration exercises.

Figure 15.2 Force plate layout with three standard plates in series and a longer plate in parallel to capture data for patients with short step length but wide base of support.

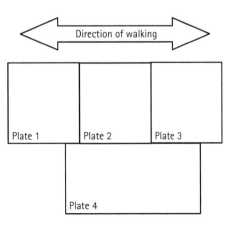

Basic principles of camera-based movement analysis systems

Overview

Most motion analysis systems are based around video camera technology. Early systems adapted cameras and other components manufactured for wider application but for the last decade cameras have been designed specifically for movement analysis. Light is supplied by light-emitting diodes (LEDs) arranged as a ring around the lens and reflects off the markers to be detected by the cameras. The LEDs function stroboscopically producing bursts of extremely high intensity and very short duration. Reflections from the markers are therefore much more intense than those arising from ambient light, which allows the sensitivity of the camera to be reduced to a level where the background appears black, but the images of the markers are preserved. The short bursts of light from the strobes reduce the overall power and can have a shuttering effect to 'freeze' images of moving markers.

The image produced by the markers within the camera is analysed to detect how many markers there are and where they are in the two-dimensional image captured by the camera. The light must have travelled from the marker in a straight line through the lens to create the image; so this information can be used to specify a *ray* from the camera along which the marker must lie. If the location of the camera and the direction in which it is pointing are known then a number of rays from each camera across the capture volume can be calculated. The process of determining the location and orientation of cameras is known as *calibration*. If a marker is seen by a number of cameras, then the respective rays from those cameras will intersect at a point and the three-dimensional coordinate of this point is taken as the marker's location (see Figure 15.3).

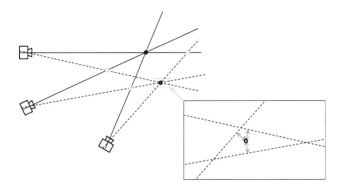

Figure 15.3 Rays from three cameras being used to reconstruct the position of two markers (black outline). Potential ghost markers (grey) occur when two rays cross at different locations. Inset gives a close-up view of one of the markers showing that the rays do not intersect exactly. The root mean square (RMS) average of the closest distance from the marker to each of the rays (grey arrows) is known as the residual.

Whilst two rays will intersect exactly in two dimensions (as in Figure 15.3), in three dimensions imperfections in the cameras and their calibration will mean that rays pass close to each other but do not intersect exactly. The inset in Figure 15.3 illustrates three rays passing close to each other but not intersecting at a single point. The (RMS) average of the closest distance from the marker to each of the rays is known as the marker *residual*. In general, the lower the residual, the closer the rays are to intersecting at a point and higher the quality of the reconstruction. Modern systems set-up for clinical gait analysis can have residuals of less than 1mm.

It is possible for two or more rays from different cameras to come close to intersecting by conicidence (grey circles in Figure 15.3), giving rise to *ghost* markers (these are less common in three dimensions than would appear from looking at such a two-dimensional representation). When many cameras are looking at many markers spaced close together then separating true from ghost markers is still a problem. Specialised software is therefore required to use the ray information to generate the coordinates of markers. This process is known as *reconstruction*. There are various strategies for identifying true marker locations. The most obvious is to impose a limit on how far a ray can pass from a proposed marker position to be assumed to be arising from it. As can be seen from Figure 15.3, real markers are seen by three cameras whereas ghost markers are only seen by two; so imposing a minimum number of cameras that detect a marker can also be useful.

Reconstruction for modern multi-camera multi-marker systems is a time-consuming process, particularly if each frame of data is handled independently. An alternative is to use data from previous frames. If there is confidence that a marker has been located correctly in one frame, then it would be expected to be close to that location in the next frame. If data from more than one earlier frame are available, then the speed and acceleration of the marker can be used to predict even more accurately where it is likely to be. Different manufacturers use different algorithms for reconstruction and also offer varying amounts of control to the user. Default settings should generally work well for routine clinical gait analysis, but developing experience in fine tuning systems may be required for specific measurement applications.

Image processing
The amount and accuracy of information captured by each camera's sensor is a key determinant of the quality of reconstruction. The amount of information is determined by both *pixel* and *grey-scale resolution* of the camera (see Figure 15.4). Pixel resolution is generally well understood. The very latest sensors have 16 million pixels (4075×3456 pixels). Many gait analysis services function well with cameras with considerably lower pixel resolutions. Grey-scale resolution is less well understood and relates to the minimal difference in light intensity that a camera can resolve. The level to which the camera can record this is often quoted and may be as high as 10 bit (1024 different levels). This may be misleading, however, as the useful resolution will be dictated by noise within the optical and electronic systems. This is exceedingly difficult to quantify and rarely quoted by manufacturers but is likely to be considerably less than the nominal grey-scale resolution.

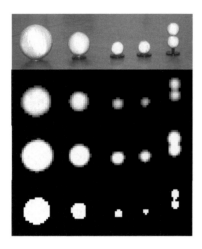

Figure 15.4 A range of markers of different diameters (50, 25 and 14mm) and the images detected by the sensor. Top image is a well-adjusted grey scale. The middle image uses grey scale but too much light is being admitted resulting in loss of grey-scale resolution from the middle of the marker. The bottom image is with threshold detection (black and white). The fourth marker from the left is older and dirtier than the third; so it gives a smaller image despite these two markers being of the same diameter.

Because of the way that information from the different pixels representing the marker is processed, the accuracy to which the centroid of the marker can be determined is considerably less than the pixel resolution of the camera and will depend on how the image is processed. Older software is based on *threshold detection*, the sensor measured whether the intensity of the light at each pixel was above or below some threshold value. Therefore in the lowest image (Figure 15.4), pixels are either black or white. Here the centroid resolution in one direction (horizontal or vertical) is inversely proportional to the number of lines of pixels across the marker image in the perpendicular direction. Therefore a marker spanning 4 pixels can be resolved twice as accurately as one spanning 2 pixels. Other than that it has a small effect on how many lines are detected as above threshold light intensity does not affect centroid resolution.

More recent systems use *grey-scale* detection, allowing the intensity of light to be measured at each pixel (see Figure 15.4, middle images). In these systems, resolution is inversely proportionate to the area of the image (rather than its diameter) *and* to the range of resolvable grey-scale levels. For a circular image 5 pixels wide, 10-level grey-scale detection will therefore give a centroid resolution of 20 times better than threshold detection, and this factor will increase with the pixel width of the marker and the number of grey-scale levels.

The dependence of centroid resolution on grey-scale levels is particularly important because it makes resolution dependent on marker illumination. A marker image that is twice as bright will have twice the number of grey-scale levels present in its image, and centroid resolution will therefore be twice as good. On the other hand, if the sensor becomes saturated (there is more light than the maximum level recordable), then the grey-scale information is effectively lost. The third row of images in Figure 15.4 shows overillumination, with grey-scale information being lost over the centre of the markers which just appear in full white. Image intensity is governed by the intensity of illumination and the camera aperture. The optical quality (particularly the depth of field) improves with smaller apertures, and if possible it is generally a good idea to use small apertures and increase the strobe intensity to achieve optimum levels of image intensity.

A further development in image processing is the use of *pattern recognition*. Given that light is being reflected off circular markers, it is relatively straightforward to predict the expected variation of light across the marker image. The measured pattern of variation can be matched to this to give even smaller centroid resolutions. It is even possible to use these techniques to detect the true centres of overlapping markers or markers that are otherwise partially occluded from a camera.

It is not just the quantity of information that is important, however, but also the quality. The camera lens introduces a distortion in which straight lines in the real world appear as curves in the captured image. This is most apparent in wide-angle and fish-eye lenses but is present to some extent in all lenses. If the characteristics of this are known, then they could be modelled in the software. An alternative is a process called *linearisation* in which correction factors are calculated from the images captured of a known object. This has the advantage of incorporating any artefacts arising from the sensor or electronics as well as the optical systems. Some manufacturers linearise cameras in the factory and others combine linearisation with camera calibration which has the advantage of being able to change lenses without requiring factory linearisation.

Grey-scale image processing and pattern recognition increases the available information by at least an order of magnitude over threshold detection and therefore offers huge potential for improvements in resolution (it is a little disappointing that mainstream manufacturers' software does not, generally, reflect this). Perhaps more importantly, the information-rich images combined with advanced linearisation techniques offer the potential for software solutions to obtain high-quality reconstruction from lower quality optical and electronic systems. This has led very recently to extremely cheap camera systems coming onto the market. Detailed comparisons with the more expensive systems have yet to be published, but early evidence suggests that these can perform excellently and may be adequate for many requirements of a basic clinical gait analysis. They have generally been developed for different markets, however, and there can be barriers to clinical use. Medical device certification may not be available. They generally do not support simultaneous capture of force plate or electromyographic data, and software for modelling and presenting data may not be readily available. Whilst still not available at the time of writing this book, there is a strong possibility of such innovations driving down the cost of movement analysis systems considerably in the near future.

Marker maintenance
Before considering camera set-up, it is worth pointing out that markers do get dirty over time as a consequence of handling and become less reflective (see Figure 15.4). This can easily be checked by moving them away from a camera and noting the distance at which they disappear. It is worth checking this distance for new markers and setting a minimum distance for markers to be considered usable. This should clearly exceed the farthest point of the measurement volume from any camera.

Camera set-up

So far, resolution has been described in terms of the pixel resolution. The absolute resolution depends on the size of object that each pixel on the sensor represents. The smaller the absolute size of the pixel, the better the absolute resolution. Good camera placement (and lens selection) is essentially the process of minimising the absolute size of pixels for each camera. A one megapixel has a sensor that is 1000 pixels across (=$\sqrt{1}$ megapixel). The width of one pixel is therefore 1000th of the horizontal distance the camera can detect (called its *linear field of view, LFOV*). Therefore, if the LFOV is 1m, then the pixel width will be 1mm. The LFOV and thus the pixel size depend on the distance from the camera. Figure 15.5 shows a 1 megapixel camera set up 4m from the centre of a 4m × 1m capture volume, with a focal length selected to just cover the width of that volume at its nearest point. The LFOV at the front of the volume is 1m (by definition), but it will be 3m at the opposite end of the capture volume. The pixel resolution therefore varies between 1 and 3mm along the capture volume and the image of a 7mm marker will vary in diameter between 7 pixels and just over 2 pixels. Variability in pixel resolution for a marker of a given diameter will therefore vary by a factor of D_F/D_N where D_F is the farthest distance from the camera and D_N is the nearest distance.

The intensity of light illuminating the marker is inversely proportional to the square of the distance from the strobe unit and the proportion of this that is detected by the sensor will be inversely proportional to the square of the distance back to the camera (the same distance), making the overall image intensity inversely proportional to the distance raised to the fourth power. Given that centroid resolution using grey-scale detection is dependent on intensity through the variation in grey-scale levels, this will vary similarly. Taking this effect and that described in the preceding paragraph together, the absolute centroid resolution for a given camera will vary with $(D_F/D_N)^5$. Therefore in the example in Figure 15.5, the absolute resolution at the farthest distance from the camera within the capture volume would be 243 times worse than that at nearest distance.

This would not be a particular problem if illumination could be optimised for markers farthest from the camera without prejudicing performance for markers closer to the

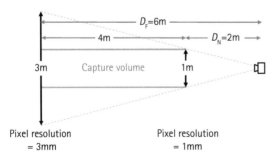

Figure 15.5 Linear field of view for a 1 megapixel camera covering a capture volume 4m long and 1m wide at a distance of 4m from its centre.

camera but as described above, overillumination leads to loss of grey-scale information through saturation. Even with threshold detection, overillumination of the closer markers, however, leads to *blooming* in which excessive brightness leads to loss of focus, increased image diameter and a potential lack of ability to distinguish between closely placed markers.

The other option is to reduce the ratio D_F/D_N. This can be reduced substantially by having the camera further away from the capture volume. Moving the camera 1m further away than in the example in Figure 15.5 will reduce the variability in absolute centroid resolution by a factor of 4 (and 2m by a factor of 8). Therefore placing the cameras as far away from the capture volume as possible will improve overall performance (as will being content with a shorter measurement volume). This is much less of an issue for cameras to the side of the capture volume as the person walks across the field of view, resulting in considerably less variation in distance from the camera. Simply moving the cameras back, whilst reducing variability in resolution, will mean that the camera LFOV is wider than necessary and will therefore 'waste' resolution. Changing to lenses of a longer focal length will enable the LFOV to be matched to the dimensions of the capture volume. Some manufacturers can supply zoom lenses, which allow continuous adjustment of focal length.

The bigger the marker, the bigger its image will be on the sensor and the higher the resolution with which its centroid can be measured. There will, however, be more chance of marker overlap, particularly if markers are placed close together as on the foot. Markers of 14mm diameter generally work well for full-body gait analysis; 9mm markers may be required for small feet. Some analysts prefer even smaller markers, but these should only be used if there is confidence that overall performance is not being affected by this.

Marker visibility and calibration

As described above, the more cameras that detect a marker the more confidence the reconstruction algorithm has that it has identified that marker. Because more information is being used to reconstruct the position of that marker, more cameras also lead to more accurate reconstructions. This accuracy is also determined by the relative placement of cameras. Figure 15.6 illustrates the general principle that cameras with a large angular separation will generally reconstruct the position of a marker better than those close together. System performance will be enhanced by ensuring that as many cameras as possible with as wide an angular separation as possible detect each marker throughout the data capture.

The other important factor is the quality of camera calibration. Most manufacturers now use a *wand calibration* in which an object (the wand) incorporating markers at known fixed distances from one another is waved in the capture volume. From this information, the software can work out where each camera must have been in order to capture the recorded images (and may also adjust linearisation parameters as well). The quality of this calibration will generally be improved by ensuring that the wand is waved through the entire calibration volume and that this covers the field

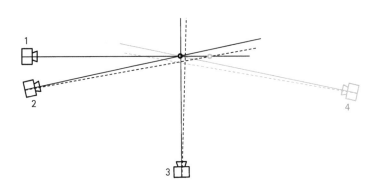

Figure 15.6 Accuracy of reconstruction from different combinations of two cameras. Solid rays give a true representation of marker position (black circle). The dashed lines show the effect of the same small error in determining the ray orientation from cameras 2 and 3. If rays from cameras close together (1 and 2) are used for reconstruction, then this has a large effect on marker location (grey circle). If rays from cameras are much further apart (1 and 2), then the effect is much smaller. Note that it is the angular separation rather than the physical separation that is important, and camera 4 gives a similar magnitude or error to camera 2.

of view of each camera. Calibration software should give feedback that this has been achieved. If waving the wand through the calibration volume does not adequately cover the field of view of the camera, it suggests that either the camera should be moved in towards the volume or preferably a longer focal length lens be used to close down the field of view. It should be noted that some metrics describing the quality of calibration may give high values if the wand is only moved a small distance in the centre of the volume. This indicates that the system is very well calibrated in the volume of the wand wave but may not be indicative of good calibration throughout the measurement volume.

Waving the wand only allows a relative camera calibration in which position and orientation of cameras in relation to each other are determined. In most clinical gait analysis, it is also necessary to know where they are in relation to the laboratory and in particular in relation to force plates. Manufacturers therefore generally allow the wand to be attached to a force plate such that the position of the wand markers in relation to the plate is known. A short data capture then allows the relative camera calibration to be aligned with a global laboratory coordinate system. There can sometimes be some variation in how the wand attaches to the plate, and in this case a visual check is essential to ensure good alignment. If the wand is used, it should be positioned centrally within the measurement volume to minimise the effect of potential errors in alignment across the volume. A much better alternative is to drill holes in the floor at precisely measured locations across the measurement volume and locate markers using these for this calibration.

Force plates

Modern force plates generally represent extremely high precision engineering. Raw force plate measurements are probably the most accurate data that are captured during the gait analysis process. Force plates are also generally quite robust instruments. The majority function for years, even decades, with little or no maintenance and no deterioration in the quality of measurements made. There are two likely causes of error (apart from accurate detection of clean foot contacts which is described in Chapter 11). The first is hardware malfunction. This can be within the force plates, cables, connectors or amplifiers. As mentioned, this is quite rare with fixed force plates but does happen occasionally. Portable or semiportable plates are more vulnerable to damage whilst being relocated, and care is also needed with connectors and cables. Particular care is required when amplifier settings are changed for a particular reason (e.g. if an adult is assessed in a centre that normally assesses children) to ensure that the original settings are restored before the resumption of routine testing.

The second probable source of error is in determining the position and orientation of the plates, which is now generally part of the calibration of the motion capture system. This generally involves a frame with markers attached being fitted to the plate in some way. There is significant variation in the way that some frames attach and it is important that local procedures specify in detail how consistent placement is to be achieved. Errors on the force plate to which the frame attaches will generally be small if reasonable care is taken. More and more services, however, are installing multiple force plates. Measurements taken on plates some distance from the one to which the frame has been fitted can be considerably more prone to error from this source. For this reason, it is sensible to apply the frame to the most central plate within the capture volume. Spot-checks are also advised as part of routine procedures (see below), but analysts should still also learn how to detect errors from review of the kinetic data (see Chapter 11).

Five steps to setting up a movement analysis laboratory

There are broadly three different ways a movement analysis laboratory can be used. Many laboratories, particularly gait laboratories, are only ever used to measure one sort of movement (walking for gait laboratories). In such laboratories, it is sensible to spend some time setting the laboratory up and then mounting cameras rigidly in given positions and using fixed focal length lenses. This minimises the potential for the configuration to be changed accidently. Many other laboratories will capture different individuals performing different movements on different days. Different calibration volumes may well be required on different occasions, and flexibility will be required in setting up the laboratory. In this case, the principles of setting the laboratory up will need to be mastered and applied on a regular basis. Cameras will generally be on tripods or other flexible mounting systems. Considerably flexibility can also be obtained by using zoom lenses. Given that set-up is regularly practised, staff can become extremely good at optimising systems to different requirements. Perhaps the most dangerous scenario is when a movement analysis laboratory is generally used for a single movement type but occasionally used for other purposes. Staff in such laboratories may well not be skilled in system set-up, and there is a great danger for mistakes to be made in setting up for the new conditions or reverting back afterwards to the usual configuration. Great care is required.

The steps required for setting up all the systems are essentially the same. In outlining the steps for setting up a movement analysis below the specific example of setting up a clinical gait analysis laboratory will be used.

1. Define the requirement
There are at least six factors that are required to define the user requirement for any particular motion capture. A typical requirement for clinical gait analysis of adults is specified on the right below.

Capture volume	3m long by 1m wide by 2m high
Task to be analysed	Walking
Preferred direction of the individual	Walking both ways along walkway
Location of markers on the individual	Conventional gait model
Any obstacles to cameras views	None
Force plates (number and location)	3 in line down centre of walkway

2. Obtain a system
It is important that this step comes after user requirements have been specified as these will dictate which system should be purchased. Broadly speaking, better systems are more expensive; so the balance is between cost and performance. If buying a system nowadays, the first step is to go for a system using full grey-scale imaging. The second is to work out, in light of the user requirement, how many cameras will be needed in order that each marker can be seen by at least three cameras throughout the task to be analysed. Eight cameras will generally provide adequate coverage for full-body analysis of walking. About 10 or 12 may be needed to obtain reliable data from multiple foot markers simultaneously. Until recently, purchasing cameras of the maximal pixel resolution possible was advisable. The most recent developments (16 megapixels) are probably beyond the requirements of most clinical services. There are similar issues with capture rate. Most current systems can capture at 100–120Hz, which is more than adequate for clinical gait analysis (although faster sample rates may be required for running).

3. Map out the capture volume
Mapping out the capture volume is extremely useful for optimising camera set-up. As a minimum, markers should be placed on the floor at the corners of the calibration volume and more centrally. Suspending markers from the ceiling can also be extremely useful for aiming cameras. Using marker pairs as on the right side of Figure 15.4 can be particularly useful. The fact that the lower grey-scale image in this figure is overilluminated is much clearer from the marker pair image, and it is otherwise impossible to gauge the size of the marker from the pixellated image (see Figure 15.7).

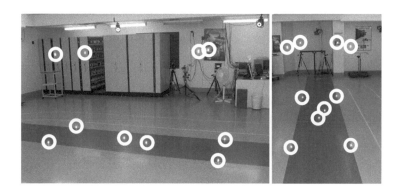

Figure 15.7 Markers mapping out the capture volume. Four are placed on the floor at corners of the volume and two more centrally. Four other markers are suspended from the ceiling at just above the head height.

4. Position cameras

Positioning eight or more modern cameras to detect a full-body marker set in a room of reasonable dimensions should be quite straightforward. Obtaining simultaneous data on multiple foot markers can be more challenging. Fewer cameras, lower resolution cameras, a smaller room, obstacles (from simple stairs or ramps to complex fluoroscopy units), or particularly close markers all make set-up much more challenging. Under these conditions, placing cameras to pick up particular movements optimally is at least as much an art as it is a science. It can require considerable trial and error and is most easily accomplished if the cameras are mounted on tripods even if the final intention is to mount them rigidly. Some manufacturers are starting to develop software to assist in choosing camera placements, but this is not yet widely available in biomechanics applications.

Following the importance of the ratio D_F/D_N for determining overall performance, all cameras should be located as far as possible from the capture volume in all but the biggest laboratories. Given this, focal lenses should be chosen such that the capture volume (as mapped out by the markers) fills the field of view of each camera. It is worth noting that modern LED strobe units have a field of illumination, which should be matched to the field of view of the camera (i.e. the focal length of the lens). It is particularly important to avoid having too small a field of illumination, which results in *vignetting* in which the markers in the centre of the field of view will be illuminated more than those around the periphery. This is a particular issue in smaller laboratories where short focal length (wide angle) lenses may be required.

An even distribution of cameras around the individual is generally optimal. In long thin laboratories, however, the front/rear cameras that are farthest from the individual may perform better than side cameras for the reasons outlined above. In this case, placing more cameras at the ends of the room may be more effective than distributing the cameras evenly. Specific movements or marker sets might require different camera placements. If viewing medial markers (medial epicondyle or malleolus) is important, then increasing the number of front/rear cameras may increase visibility. Viewing around objects can also be difficult. In either of these cases, placing cameras quite close together can appear sensible, but it should be remembered that reconstruction accuracy is reduced if the angle between rays used in the reconstruction is small.

Although theoretically reconstruction would be optimised by having cameras at a range of heights, practical concerns generally dictate the height of cameras. Having them high up generally keeps them out of the way and allows them to see over furniture or people around the periphery of the laboratory. If all cameras are pointing down slightly then there is little chance of the strobe output of one camera affecting the performance of the opposite camera either directly or through reflection off the floor. Occasionally this cannot be avoided in which case use of non-reflective floor covering or even ensuring that opposing cameras are operating in different parts of the spectrum, so a visible red strobe and filter is used on one camera and infra-red on the opposing camera may be useful.

5. Tune cameras

The amount of adjustment that is available will depend on individual cameras and measurement systems but is likely to include focus, aperture, strobe intensity and sensor gain and threshold. In movement analysis, the front focus is generally set to infinity and locked to ensure that this setting is not lost accidently. Locking the front focus makes the cameras susceptible to the quality of the back focus (the extent to which the lens is screwed into the casing). Occasionally, particularly if lenses are swapped frequently, it may be necessary to adjust this. Periodic checks of focus (perhaps every few months or if a drop in reconstruction quality is suspected) are sensible. Adjusting focus based on spherical marker images is difficult, and making a more complex image out of strips of retroreflective tape stuck to cardboard can be very useful.

Aperture, gain and strobe intensity all effectively change the intensity of the image created by the camera The overall aim is to ensure maximum grey-scale information for all markers across the measurement volume. This requires adjusting these settings so that as many pixels as possible are detected for each marker but that as few of these pixels as possible are saturated. As with all optical systems, increasing the aperture will reduce the depth of field (the ability to have markers at the front and back of the measurement volume in focus at the same time). The grey-scale resolution is effectively limited by the system noise, which will be increased if system gain is increased. Image intensity is therefore best controlled by strobe illumination. Ideal illumination would have a good range of grey scales for the distant markers without saturation of the near markers. It is extremely unlikely that this can be achieved for cameras viewing along the capture volume. Given that saturation is likely to affect the images of markers closer to the camera which will also cover a larger number of pixels and therefore generally have good centroid resolution, this may need to be tolerated to ensure adequate illumination of distant markers.

A threshold is applied to remove low-level noise across the sensor and helps with image processing. It needs to be remembered that centroid resolution is dependent on the range of grey-scale levels available. Only the minimal threshold required to remove the noise should be used otherwise the number of grey-scale levels may be reduced unnecessarily. For this reason, it is not generally a good idea to remove reflections from opposing cameras by increasing the threshold. It is far better to remove these by adjusting camera positions or other means.

Note that some modern systems operating in real time make compromises in signal processing to do so. For example, full grey-scale detection or pattern recognition techniques may not be used in real time but may apply to postprocessing of data. It is important that the user of the system understands differences in these two processes and optimises the camera set-up for the processing that will actually be used. In most clinical gait analysis, for example, this will be the full postprocessing option.

Maintaining a motion analysis laboratory

Modern motion capture systems require little maintenance and can function for years without faults developing. Because of the complexity of measurements, however, when faults do develop they can easily go undetected and some vigilance is required. Manufacturers generally provide measures of system performance, but these are generally not useful for routine biomechanical interpretation and can be disregarded. The marker residuals are a measure of how close rays from different cameras attributable to an individual marker come to intersecting. Calibration residuals describe how closely rays from the same camera come to the calculated marker positions. Acceptable levels for both should be set for each installation and monitored to ensure adequate system performance. Some manufacturers also feedback the calculated distance between the markers on the calibration wand as another check on performance. General performance of marker calibration, reconstruction, tracking and autolabelling are also indicators of overall data quality. Performance of these should be monitored and any deterioration in performance should be investigated. It should be noted that most modern systems perform extremely well for clinical gait analysis. If problems are encountered in any of these aspects of performance, then it suggests that the system has not been set up properly.

Perhaps the one item of gait analysis equipment that does deteriorate in performance is the marker. These accumulate dirt over time. If system performance is noticed to be falling, then checking the markers is indicated. Place them on the floor beyond the farthest corner of the capture volume from any camera and ensure that they can be seen by that relevant camera. They can be washed in mild detergent but do need to be replaced every so often – perhaps after somewhere between 50 and 100 gait analyses. They do seem expensive for what they are and some laboratories are reluctant to replace them, but given the overall costs of delivering a clinical gait analysis service it is ridiculous to jeopardise the quality of measurements for such a relatively small expense. (It is possible to recover the markers but this is so time consuming that it almost certainly costs more in labour costs than simply paying for replacements.)

The most probable errors to arise are through intentional or inadvertent adjustment of settings. Having these saved as defaults in the software and re-applied at the start of each capture session can protect against this to a certain extent. It can also be useful to perform occasional spot-checks on system performance. How often to do this depends a little on patient throughput. Mapping out the capture volume and checking settings is quite easy to perform. The most modern systems employing pattern recognition can resolve closely packed markers (e.g. ten 14mm markers arranged in a close packed triangle like the red balls at the start of a snooker match) when set up optimally. Testing the system in this way is a good way to ensure that the system is performing optimally. SAMSA (Piazza et al. 2007) is a device in which a motor rotates a metal bar on which markers are mounted, some of which are masked from various cameras. Various metrics by which system accuracy can be assessed are defined. It has been designed as a standard for assessing marker location accuracy and can be a useful spot-check on system performance as well.

Another test uses a poker to test the agreement of kinematic and kinetic measuring systems (Holden 2003) (Figure 15.8). As the load is applied through the top and bottom tips of the poker, the ground reaction must pass through both and therefore along the length of the poker (the mass and inertia of the rod can be compensated for if required). In an ideal system, the line of the ground reaction will therefore pass along the line of the poker, which is also measured kinematically from the markers attached to it. Most gait analysis software allows a visual check that the ground reaction and poker are collinear, and a number of parameters have also been suggested to quantify

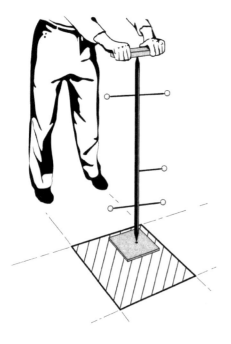

Figure 15.8 A rigid mechanical device being used to apply forces to the force plate (Figure from Holden 2003 with permission).

this. There have been several suggestions to go one stage further and propose methods for in situ calibration of force plates (Chiari et al. 2000; Cappello et al. 2004; Collins et al. 2009). Modern force plates are precision engineered with factory-based calibration to high levels of accuracy. Considerable confidence in in situ calibration techniques is required to override the results of such a process, and the option of returning a plate for repeat factory calibration should always be considered if the calibration is considered to be poor.

In conclusion, setting up and maintaining a gait analysis laboratory is a reasonably complex process. Whilst manufacturers will often install equipment on behalf of clients such that it can be operated by people with no specific technical knowledge, there is a strong possibility that such set-up will not be optimised to the users' requirements and a risk of problems developing and going undetected with equipment. If clinical decisions are being made on the basis of measurements made by such equipment, there is a strong argument that this risk should be classified as unacceptable. Obtaining external advice on laboratory design, construction and maintenance is not easy, and the solution adopted by most leading centres is to ensure that at least one senior staff member has the competencies to ensure the quality of system maintenance and ongoing performance.

References

Cappello A, Lenzi D, Chiari L. Periodical in-situ re-calibration of force platforms: a new method for the robust estimation of the calibration matrix. *Med Biol Eng Comput*, 2004, 42:350–355.

Chiari L, Cappello A, Lenzi D, Della Croce U. An improved technique for the extraction of stochastic parameters from stabilograms. *Gait Posture*, 2000, 12:225–234.

Collins SH, Adamczyk PG, Ferris DP, Kuo AD. A simple method for calibrating force plates and force treadmills using an instrumented pole. *Gait Posture*, 2009, 29:59–64. DOI: 10.1016/j.gaitpost.2008.06.010

Holden J. A proposed test to support the clinical movement analysis laboratory accreditation process. *Gait Posture*, 2003, 17:205–213.

Piazza SJ, Chou L-S, Denniston N et al. A proposed standard for assessing the marker-location accuracy of video-based motion analysis systems. In: *12th Annual Meeting of the Gait and Clinical Movement Analysis Society*, Springfield, MA, 2007.

Appendix 1: Limitations of the conventional subdivision of the gait cycle

Although almost all text books on clinical gait analysis recommend one particular subdivision of the gait cycle into phases (Perry 1992) there are some problems associated with it. *Initial contact* is clearly an instant and not a phase, and we already have a term for it (foot contact). *Response* implies something that occurs after an event. It is clear from the most cursory inspection of the vertical component of the ground reaction that loading occurs throughout first single support and that *loading response* is therefore not a particularly well-chosen term for this phase (see Figure A1.1). *Mid-stance* does not occur in the middle of stance and *terminal stance* does not occur at the end of it.

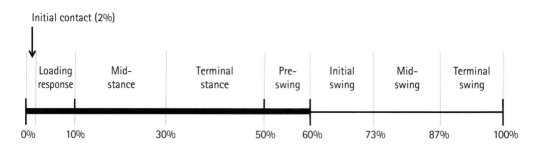

Figure A1.1 Phases of the gait cycle as defined by Perry (1992). Timings refer to normal walking only.

There is a particular issue here with many clinicians who have not been influenced by instrumented gait analysis using mid-stance to refer to the middle of stance and terminal stance to refer to the end of stance, whereas those who have been trained in instrumented gait analysis will tend to use these more formal definitions. Some people do not like *pre-swing* being a phase of stance, but this does reinforce the cyclic nature of walking and that one of the most important functions in late stance is to prepare for swing. It may well be, using the same reasoning, that *pre-stance* is a good alternative term for terminal swing.

A further issue is that in order to correlate what is happening on one side to what is happening on the other at the same phase in gait, it would have been useful if single support and swing (being the same phases of gait but observed with regard to different limbs) had been subdivided into the same number of subphases.

The precise way the transitions between the subphases of single support and swing is determined in terms of characteristics of healthy walking and often does not translate well to other walking patterns. Terminal stance, for example, is defined as commencing with heel rise, which is not meaningful in some patients who never achieve heel contact. Similarly mid-swing ends with tibia vertical, which may never occur in people who walk with a crouch gait pattern.

Reference
Perry J. *Gait Analysis.* Thorofare, NJ, SLACK, 1992.

Appendix 2: Other measures of repeatability

There are a number of different techniques for quantifying repeatability that have been used in previous studies. These often express the variability as a ratio of another quantity and are expressed as either a percentage or an index with a value between 0 and 1. Whilst these are generally equally valid statistically, there are at least three challenges in understanding how to use the results in relation to the interpretation of clinical data The most obvious is that the index gives no indication of the actual magnitude of variability. The second is that they do not report measurement variability alone but variability in relation to something else and can produce misleading results unless this process is fully understood (examples are given below). Finally they are often characterised by descriptors that have been developed in different contexts and can be highly misleading in relation to gait data (see comments in relation to the ICC below).

Coefficient of variation

The *coefficient of variation* (CV) is the standard deviation of a measurement divided by its mean value (or sometimes the mean absolute value) (Winter 2009) and expressed as a percentage. Issues with its use are illustrated in Table A2.1. In this example, there is similar absolute variability in pelvic tilt, hip flexion and knee flexion but considerably different values of the coefficient of variation because the mean values for these angles throughout the gait cycle are different. There is a particular issue for dorsiflexion where the average value is quite close to zero and absolute variability which is half that in the other variables results in a coefficient of variation which is over three times as big. Comparison of the CV can thus give quite mis-leading impression of the relative reapatability of the different measures.

Table A2.1 Calculation of the coefficient of variability from sagittal plane data

Variable	Variability (SD)	Mean	Coefficient of variation (%)
Pelvic tilt	4°	31°	31
Hip flexion	4°	18°	22
Knee flexion	4°	24°	17
Ankle dorsiflexion	2°	2°	100

Coefficient of multiple correlation

The *coefficient of multiple correlation* (CMC) was introduced into repeatability studies of gait analysis by Kadaba et al. (1989). It is the square root of the coefficient of multiple determination (CMD), which is effectively one minus the ratio of the variance between gait cycles divided by the total variance including that across the gait cycles.

$$CMD = 1 - \frac{\sigma^2_{between\,cycles}}{\sigma^2_{total\,across\,cycles}}$$

This has exactly the same limitations as the coefficient of variation in that it depends on the magnitude to the total variance. Indicative values are given in Table A2.2, which indicates how the relatively small range of pelvic tilt throughout the gait cycle results in a low CMC regardless of the fact that the absolute variability is no worse than that for the hip or knee. It should also be noted that the particular manner in which the CMC

Table A2.2 Calculation of the coefficient of multiple correlation from sagittal plane data

Variable	Variability (between cycles, SD)	Variability (within cycle, SD)	CMC
Pelvic tilt	4°	0.6°	0.39
Hip flexion	4°	16°	0.98
Knee flexion	4°	17°	0.99
Ankle dorsiflexion	2°	8°	0.98

is defined can give results very close to one even when there is appreciable absolute variability. Although there is half the absolute variability at the ankle in Table A2.2, the CMC is 1% worse than for the knee.

Intraclass correlation coefficient

The *intraclass correlation coefficient* (ICC) is also a variance ratio for a sample of individuals. It is defined as the ratio of the 'true' variance (between individuals) to the total variance (including measurement variability) (Portney and Watkins 2009). It has similar limitations to the other two ratios discussed above. A further issue is that the ratio will depend on the characteristics of the sample chosen for the repeatability study. Therefore if the study involves patients with a large number of gait patterns, the resulting ICC will be higher than a study involving healthy individuals with very similar gait patterns. There are at least three variants of the ICC (Shrout and Fleiss 1979) that result in quite different values for the same datasets. Many studies do not report which version was used (McGinley et al. 2009). Finally the ICC was first applied in psychology for fairly 'soft' measurement instruments where low levels of agreement were much more acceptable than in clinical gait analysis. An early paper (Landis and Koch 1977) suggested that values of the ICC as low as 0.6 should be regarded as indicating 'substantial' agreement and over 0.8 as 'almost perfect'. More recent texts are less generous with Portney and Watkins, suggesting that 'for many clinical measurements, reliability should exceed 0.9 to ensure reasonable validity' (Portney and Watkins 2009).

Ad hoc methods

The study of Noonan et al. (2003) caused considerable consternation within the gait analysis community when the results were first announced (Gage 2003; Wright 2003). This was at least in part because they devised their own methods to analyse their repeatability studies that had little statistical justification and included a measure they called the *discordance index*. This index focused on the range of measurements rather than the standard deviation and tended to exaggerate the variability within measurements.

Whilst the gait analysis community is generally correct to point out that these measures tend to exaggerate variability, it is also salient to remember that a single standard deviation tends to underrepresent the variability. By definition, over a third of measurements will be more than one standard deviation away from the mean value.

References

Gage J. Con: Interobserver variability of gait analysis. *Journal of Pediatric Orthopaedics*, 2003, 23:290–291.

Kadaba MP, Ramakrishnan HK, Wootten ME, Gainey J, Gorton G, Cochran GV. Repeatability of kinematic, kinetic, and electromyographic data in normal adult gait. *J Orthop Res*, 1989, 7:849–860. DOI: 10.1002/jor.1100070611

Landis JR, Koch GG. The measurement of observer agreement for categorical data. *Biometrics*, 1977, 33:159–174. DOI: 10.2307/2529310

McGinley JL, Baker R, Wolfe R, Morris ME. The reliability of three–dimensional kinematic gait measurements: a systematic review. *Gait Posture*, 2009, 29:360–369. DOI: 10.1016/j.gaitpost.2008.09.003

Noonan K, Halliday S, Browne R, O'Brien S, Kayes K, Feinberg J. Inter-observer variability of gait analysis in patients with cerebral palsy. *J Pediatr Orthop*, 2003, 23:279–287.

Portney LG, Watkins MP. *Foundations of Clinical Research: Applications to Practice.* Prentice-Hall, Upper Saddle River, NJ, 2009.

Shrout PE, Fleiss JL. Intra-class correlations: uses in assessing rater reliability. *Psychol Bull*, 1979, 86:420–428. DOI: 10.1037/0033-2909.86.2.420

Winter DA. *Biomechanics and Motor Control or Human Movement.* John Wiley and Sons, Hoboken, NJ, 2009.

Wright J. Pro: Interobserver variability of Gait Analysis. *J Pediatr Orthop*, 2003, 23:288–289.

Index

Index

Index

Index